50% OFF
Online CPHQ Prep Course!

Dear Customer,

Thank you for your purchase of this CPHQ Study Guide. Included with your purchase is **discounted access to our online CPHQ Prep Course.** Many CPHQ courses cost hundreds of dollars and don't deliver enough value. Our course provides the best CPHQ prep material, and with discounted access, **you only pay half price**.

We have structured our online course to perfectly complement your printed study guide. The CPHQ Prep Course contains **in-depth lessons** that cover all the most important topics, over **950 practice questions** to ensure you feel prepared, and more than **500 digital flashcards**, so you can study while you're on the go.

Online CPHQ Prep Course

Topics Covered:

- Quality Leadership and Integration
- Performance and Process Improvement
- Population Health and Care Transitions
- Health Data Analytics
- Patient Safety
- Quality Review and Accountability
- Regulatory and Accreditation

Course Features:

- CPHQ Study Guide
  - Get content that complements our best-selling study guide.
- Full-Length Practice Tests
  - With over 950 practice questions, you can test yourself again and again.
- Mobile Friendly
  - If you need to study on the go, the course is easily accessible from your mobile device.
- CPHQ Flashcards
  - Our course includes a flashcard mode consisting of over 500 content cards to help you study.

To lock in your discounted access, visit mometrix.com/university/cphq or simply scan this QR code with your smartphone. At the checkout page, enter the discount code: **cphq50off**

If you have any questions or concerns, please contact us at support@mometrix.com.

Sincerely,

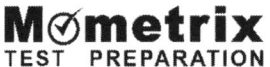

Access Your Online Resources

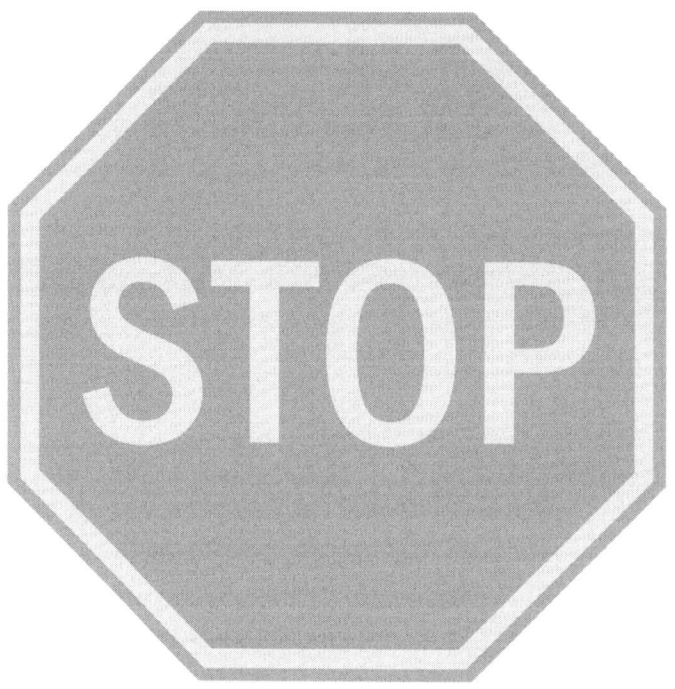

Don't miss out on the Online Resources included with your purchase!

Your purchase of this product unlocks access to our Online Resources page. Elevate your study experience with our **interactive practice test interface**, along with all of the additional resources that we couldn't include in this book.

Flip to the Online Resources section at the end of this book to find the link and a QR code to get started!

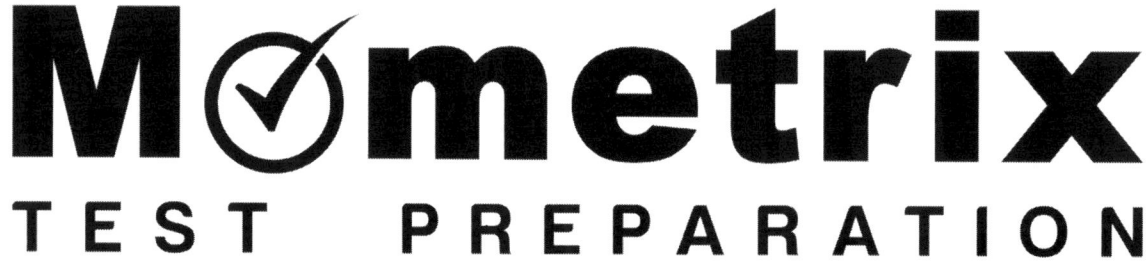

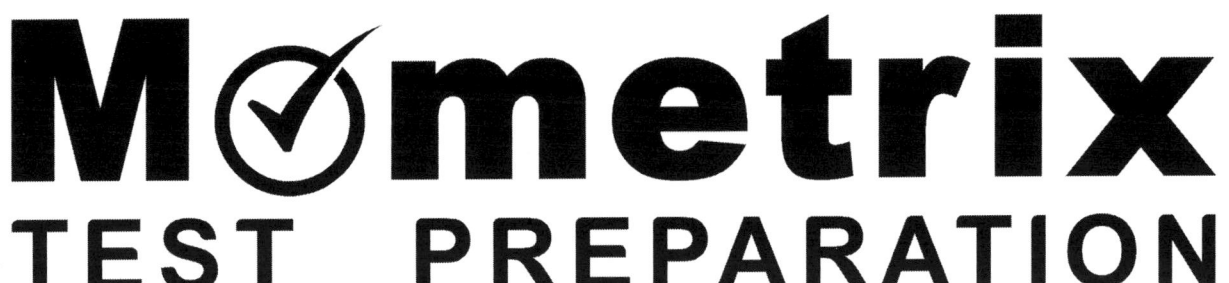

CPHQ®

Study Guide 2026-2027

4 Full-Length Practice Tests

Exam Secrets Prep Book for the NAHQ Certified Professional in Healthcare Quality®
[5th Edition]

Includes Audiobook

Copyright © 2026 by Mometrix Media LLC

All rights reserved. This product, or parts thereof, may not be reproduced, stored in a retrieval system, or transmitted in any form or by any means—electronic, mechanical, photocopy, recording, scanning, or other—except for brief quotations in critical reviews or articles, without the prior written permission of the publisher.

Written and edited by Matthew Bowling

Printed in the United States of America

This paper meets the requirements of ANSI/NISO Z39.48-1992 (Permanence of Paper).

Mometrix offers volume discount pricing to institutions. For more information or a price quote, please contact our sales department at sales@mometrix.com or 888-248-1219.

CPHQ and Certified Professional in Healthcare Quality are registered trademarks of National Association for Healthcare Quality, which is not affiliated with Mometrix Test Preparation and does not endorse this product.

Paperback
ISBN 13: 978-1-5167-2731-5
ISBN 10: 1-5167-2731-2

DEAR FUTURE EXAM SUCCESS STORY

First of all, **THANK YOU** for purchasing Mometrix study materials!

Second, congratulations! You are one of the few determined test-takers who are committed to doing whatever it takes to excel on your exam. **You have come to the right place.** We developed these study materials with one goal in mind: to deliver you the information you need in a format that's concise and easy to use.

In addition to optimizing your guide for the content of the test, we've outlined our recommended steps for breaking down the preparation process into small, attainable goals so you can make sure you stay on track.

We've also analyzed the entire test-taking process, identifying the most common pitfalls and showing how you can overcome them and be ready for any curveball the test throws you.

Standardized testing is one of the biggest obstacles on your road to success, which only increases the importance of doing well in the high-pressure, high-stakes environment of test day. Your results on this test could have a significant impact on your future, and this guide provides the information and practical advice to help you achieve your full potential on test day.

Your success is our success

We would love to hear from you! If you would like to share the story of your exam success or if you have any questions or comments in regard to our products, please contact us at **800-673-8175** or **support@mometrix.com**.

Thanks again for your business and we wish you continued success!

Sincerely,
The Mometrix Test Preparation Team

Need more help? Check out our flashcards at:
http://MometrixFlashcards.com/CPHQ

TABLE OF CONTENTS

INTRODUCTION 1
SECRET KEY #1 – PLAN BIG, STUDY SMALL 2
SECRET KEY #2 – MAKE YOUR STUDYING COUNT 3
SECRET KEY #3 – PRACTICE THE RIGHT WAY 4
SECRET KEY #4 – PACE YOURSELF 6
SECRET KEY #5 – HAVE A PLAN FOR GUESSING 7
TEST-TAKING STRATEGIES 10
FIVE-WEEK CPHQ STUDY PLAN 14
    WEEK 1: QUALITY LEADERSHIP AND INTEGRATION & QUALITY REVIEW AND ACCOUNTABILITY ... 15
    WEEK 2: PERFORMANCE AND PROCESS IMPROVEMENT 16
    WEEK 3: POPULATION HEALTH AND CARE TRANSITIONS & HEALTH DATA ANALYTICS 17
    WEEK 4: PATIENT SAFETY & REGULATORY AND ACCREDITATION 18
    WEEK 5: PRACTICE TESTS 19
QUALITY LEADERSHIP AND INTEGRATION 21
    STRATEGIC PLANNING 21
    STAKEHOLDER ENGAGEMENT 33
PERFORMANCE AND PROCESS IMPROVEMENT 36
    QUALITY IMPROVEMENT TRAINING 36
    COMMUNICATION 52
    TEAMS 55
    EVIDENCE-BASED PRACTICE 62
    LEADING AND FACILITATING CHANGE 63
    PERFORMANCE IMPROVEMENT METHODS 72
    QUALITY TOOLS AND TECHNIQUES 78
    MONITORING TIMELINESS 83
    EVALUATING EFFECTIVENESS 84
POPULATION HEALTH AND CARE TRANSITIONS 86
    POPULATION HEALTH 86
    CARE TRANSITIONS 90
HEALTH DATA ANALYTICS 92
    DATA MANAGEMENT SYSTEMS 92
    MEASUREMENT AND ANALYSIS 104
PATIENT SAFETY 123
    PATIENT RIGHTS AND PATIENT ADVOCACY 123
    TECHNOLOGY SOLUTIONS TO ENHANCE PATIENT SAFETY 127
    ENHANCING THE CULTURE OF PATIENT SAFETY 130
    SAFETY CONCEPTS 133
    SAFETY PRINCIPLES 147
    SAFETY REVIEWS 152

Quality Review and Accountability _____ 156
Standards and Best Practices _____ 156
Evaluating Compliance with Internal and External Requirements _____ 158
Maintaining Confidentiality _____ 176

Regulatory and Accreditation _____ 177
Accreditation, Certification, and Recognition Options _____ 177
Evaluating Compliance _____ 184
Survey Readiness _____ 185

CPHQ Practice Test #1 _____ 188

Answer Key and Explanations for Test #1 _____ 211

CPHQ Practice Tests #2, #3 and #4 _____ 231

How to Overcome Test Anxiety _____ 232

Online Resources _____ 238

Introduction

Thank you for purchasing this resource! You have made the choice to prepare yourself for a test that could have a huge impact on your future, and this guide is designed to help you be fully ready for test day. Obviously, it's important to have a solid understanding of the test material, but you also need to be prepared for the unique environment and stressors of the test, so that you can perform to the best of your abilities.

For this purpose, the first section that appears in this guide is the **Secret Keys**. We've devoted countless hours to meticulously researching what works and what doesn't, and we've boiled down our findings to the five most impactful steps you can take to improve your performance on the test. We start at the beginning with study planning and move through the preparation process, all the way to the testing strategies that will help you get the most out of what you know when you're finally sitting in front of the test.

We recommend that you start preparing for your test as far in advance as possible. However, if you've bought this guide as a last-minute study resource and only have a few days before your test, we recommend that you skip over the first two Secret Keys since they address a long-term study plan.

If you struggle with **test anxiety**, we strongly encourage you to check out our recommendations for how you can overcome it. Test anxiety is a formidable foe, but it can be beaten, and we want to make sure you have the tools you need to defeat it.

Secret Key #1 – Plan Big, Study Small

There's a lot riding on your performance. If you want to ace this test, you're going to need to keep your skills sharp and the material fresh in your mind. You need a plan that lets you review everything you need to know while still fitting in your schedule. We'll break this strategy down into three categories.

Information Organization

Start with the information you already have: the official test outline. From this, you can make a complete list of all the concepts you need to cover before the test. Organize these concepts into groups that can be studied together, and create a list of any related vocabulary you need to learn so you can brush up on any difficult terms. You'll want to keep this vocabulary list handy once you actually start studying since you may need to add to it along the way.

Time Management

Once you have your set of study concepts, decide how to spread them out over the time you have left before the test. Break your study plan into small, clear goals so you have a manageable task for each day and know exactly what you're doing. Then just focus on one small step at a time. When you manage your time this way, you don't need to spend hours at a time studying. Studying a small block of content for a short period each day helps you retain information better and avoid stressing over how much you have left to do. You can relax knowing that you have a plan to cover everything in time. In order for this strategy to be effective though, you have to start studying early and stick to your schedule. Avoid the exhaustion and futility that comes from last-minute cramming!

Study Environment

The environment you study in has a big impact on your learning. Studying in a coffee shop, while probably more enjoyable, is not likely to be as fruitful as studying in a quiet room. It's important to keep distractions to a minimum. You're only planning to study for a short block of time, so make the most of it. Don't pause to check your phone or get up to find a snack. It's also important to **avoid multitasking**. Research has consistently shown that multitasking will make your studying dramatically less effective. Your study area should also be comfortable and well-lit so you don't have the distraction of straining your eyes or sitting on an uncomfortable chair.

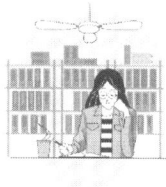

The time of day you study is also important. You want to be rested and alert. Don't wait until just before bedtime. Study when you'll be most likely to comprehend and remember. Even better, if you know what time of day your test will be, set that time aside for study. That way your brain will be used to working on that subject at that specific time and you'll have a better chance of recalling information.

Finally, it can be helpful to team up with others who are studying for the same test. Your actual studying should be done in as isolated an environment as possible, but the work of organizing the information and setting up the study plan can be divided up. In between study sessions, you can discuss with your teammates the concepts that you're all studying and quiz each other on the details. Just be sure that your teammates are as serious about the test as you are. If you find that your study time is being replaced with social time, you might need to find a new team.

Secret Key #2 – Make Your Studying Count

You're devoting a lot of time and effort to preparing for this test, so you want to be absolutely certain it will pay off. This means doing more than just reading the content and hoping you can remember it on test day. It's important to make every minute of study count. There are two main areas you can focus on to make your studying count.

Retention

It doesn't matter how much time you study if you can't remember the material. You need to make sure you are retaining the concepts. To check your retention of the information you're learning, try recalling it at later times with minimal prompting. Try carrying around flashcards and glance at one or two from time to time or ask a friend who's also studying for the test to quiz you.

To enhance your retention, look for ways to put the information into practice so that you can apply it rather than simply recalling it. If you're using the information in practical ways, it will be much easier to remember. Similarly, it helps to solidify a concept in your mind if you're not only reading it to yourself but also explaining it to someone else. Ask a friend to let you teach them about a concept you're a little shaky on (or speak aloud to an imaginary audience if necessary). As you try to summarize, define, give examples, and answer your friend's questions, you'll understand the concepts better and they will stay with you longer. Finally, step back for a big picture view and ask yourself how each piece of information fits with the whole subject. When you link the different concepts together and see them working together as a whole, it's easier to remember the individual components.

Finally, practice showing your work on any multi-step problems, even if you're just studying. Writing out each step you take to solve a problem will help solidify the process in your mind, and you'll be more likely to remember it during the test.

Modality

Modality simply refers to the means or method by which you study. Choosing a study modality that fits your own individual learning style is crucial. No two people learn best in exactly the same way, so it's important to know your strengths and use them to your advantage.

For example, if you learn best by visualization, focus on visualizing a concept in your mind and draw an image or a diagram. Try color-coding your notes, illustrating them, or creating symbols that will trigger your mind to recall a learned concept. If you learn best by hearing or discussing information, find a study partner who learns the same way or read aloud to yourself. Think about how to put the information in your own words. Imagine that you are giving a lecture on the topic and record yourself so you can listen to it later.

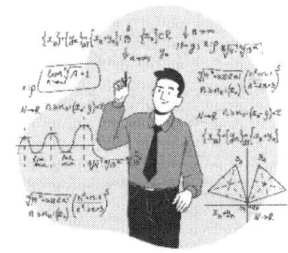

For any learning style, flashcards can be helpful. Organize the information so you can take advantage of spare moments to review. Underline key words or phrases. Use different colors for different categories. Mnemonic devices (such as creating a short list in which every item starts with the same letter) can also help with retention. Find what works best for you and use it to store the information in your mind most effectively and easily.

Secret Key #3 – Practice the Right Way

Your success on test day depends not only on how many hours you put into preparing, but also on whether you prepared the right way. It's good to check along the way to see if your studying is paying off. One of the most effective ways to do this is by taking practice tests to evaluate your progress. Practice tests are useful because they show exactly where you need to improve. Every time you take a practice test, pay special attention to these three groups of questions:

- The questions you got wrong
- The questions you had to guess on, even if you guessed right
- The questions you found difficult or slow to work through

This will show you exactly what your weak areas are, and where you need to devote more study time. Ask yourself why each of these questions gave you trouble. Was it because you didn't understand the material? Was it because you didn't remember the vocabulary? Do you need more repetitions on this type of question to build speed and confidence? Dig into those questions and figure out how you can strengthen your weak areas as you go back to review the material.

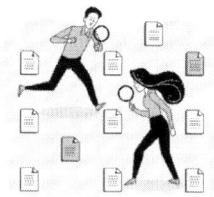

Additionally, many practice tests have a section explaining the answer choices. It can be tempting to read the explanation and think that you now have a good understanding of the concept. However, an explanation likely only covers part of the question's broader context. Even if the explanation makes perfect sense, **go back and investigate** every concept related to the question until you're positive you have a thorough understanding.

As you go along, keep in mind that the practice test is just that: practice. Memorizing these questions and answers will not be very helpful on the actual test because it is unlikely to have any of the same exact questions. If you only know the right answers to the sample questions, you won't be prepared for the real thing. **Study the concepts** until you understand them fully, and then you'll be able to answer any question that shows up on the test.

It's important to wait on the practice tests until you're ready. If you take a test on your first day of study, you may be overwhelmed by the amount of material covered and how much you need to learn. Work up to it gradually.

On test day, you'll need to be prepared for answering questions, managing your time, and using the test-taking strategies you've learned. It's a lot to balance, like a mental marathon that will have a big impact on your future. Like training for a marathon, you'll need to start slowly and work your way up. When test day arrives, you'll be ready.

Start with the strategies you've read in the first two Secret Keys—plan your course and study in the way that works best for you. If you have time, consider using multiple study resources to get different approaches to the same concepts. It can be helpful to see difficult concepts from more than one angle. Then find a good source for practice tests. Many times, the test website will suggest potential study resources or provide sample tests.

Practice Test Strategy

If you're able to find at least three practice tests, we recommend this strategy:

Untimed and Open-Book Practice

Take the first test with no time constraints and with your notes and study guide handy. Take your time and focus on applying the strategies you've learned.

Timed and Open-Book Practice

Take the second practice test open-book as well, but set a timer and practice pacing yourself to finish in time.

Timed and Closed-Book Practice

Take any other practice tests as if it were test day. Set a timer and put away your study materials. Sit at a table or desk in a quiet room, imagine yourself at the testing center, and answer questions as quickly and accurately as possible.

Keep repeating timed and closed-book tests on a regular basis until you run out of practice tests or it's time for the actual test. Your mind will be ready for the schedule and stress of test day, and you'll be able to focus on recalling the material you've learned.

Secret Key #4 – Pace Yourself

Once you're fully prepared for the material on the test, your biggest challenge on test day will be managing your time. Just knowing that the clock is ticking can make you panic even if you have plenty of time left. Work on pacing yourself so you can build confidence against the time constraints of the exam. Pacing is a difficult skill to master, especially in a high-pressure environment, so **practice is vital**.

Set time expectations for your pace based on how much time is available. For example, if a section has 60 questions and the time limit is 30 minutes, you know you have to average 30 seconds or less per question in order to answer them all. Although 30 seconds is the hard limit, set 25 seconds per question as your goal, so you reserve extra time to spend on harder questions. When you budget extra time for the harder questions, you no longer have any reason to stress when those questions take longer to answer.

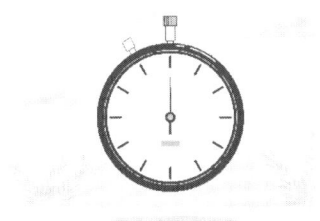

Don't let this time expectation distract you from working through the test at a calm, steady pace, but keep it in mind so you don't spend too much time on any one question. Recognize that taking extra time on one question you don't understand may keep you from answering two that you do understand later in the test. If your time limit for a question is up and you're still not sure of the answer, mark it and move on, and come back to it later if the time and the test format allow. If the testing format doesn't allow you to return to earlier questions, just make an educated guess; then put it out of your mind and move on.

On the easier questions, be careful not to rush. It may seem wise to hurry through them so you have more time for the challenging ones, but it's not worth missing one if you know the concept and just didn't take the time to read the question fully. Work efficiently but make sure you understand the question and have looked at all of the answer choices, since more than one may seem right at first.

Even if you're paying attention to the time, you may find yourself a little behind at some point. You should speed up to get back on track, but do so wisely. Don't panic; just take a few seconds less on each question until you're caught up. Don't guess without thinking, but do look through the answer choices and eliminate any you know are wrong. If you can get down to two choices, it is often worthwhile to guess from those. Once you've chosen an answer, move on and don't dwell on any that you skipped or had to hurry through. If a question was taking too long, chances are it was one of the harder ones, so you weren't as likely to get it right anyway.

On the other hand, if you find yourself getting ahead of schedule, it may be beneficial to slow down a little. The more quickly you work, the more likely you are to make a careless mistake that will affect your score. You've budgeted time for each question, so don't be afraid to spend that time. Practice an efficient but careful pace to get the most out of the time you have.

Secret Key #5 – Have a Plan for Guessing

When you're taking the test, you may find yourself stuck on a question. Some of the answer choices seem better than others, but you don't see the one answer choice that is obviously correct. What do you do?

The scenario described above is very common, yet most test takers have not effectively prepared for it. Developing and practicing a plan for guessing may be one of the single most effective uses of your time as you get ready for the exam.

In developing your plan for guessing, there are three questions to address:

- When should you start the guessing process?
- How should you narrow down the choices?
- Which answer should you choose?

When to Start the Guessing Process

Unless your plan for guessing is to select C every time (which, despite its merits, is not what we recommend), you need to leave yourself enough time to apply your answer elimination strategies. Since you have a limited amount of time for each question, that means that if you're going to give yourself the best shot at guessing correctly, you have to decide quickly whether or not you will guess.

Of course, the best-case scenario is that you don't have to guess at all, so first, see if you can answer the question based on your knowledge of the subject and basic reasoning skills. Focus on the key words in the question and try to jog your memory of related topics. Give yourself a chance to bring the knowledge to mind, but once you realize that you don't have (or you can't access) the knowledge you need to answer the question, it's time to start the guessing process.

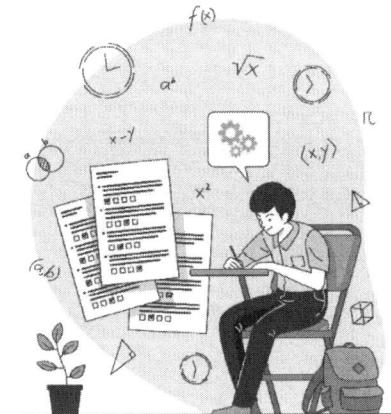

It's almost always better to start the guessing process too early than too late. It only takes a few seconds to remember something and answer the question from knowledge. Carefully eliminating wrong answer choices takes longer. Plus, going through the process of eliminating answer choices can actually help jog your memory.

Summary: Start the guessing process as soon as you decide that you can't answer the question based on your knowledge.

How to Narrow Down the Choices

The next chapter in this book (**Test-Taking Strategies**) includes a wide range of strategies for how to approach questions and how to look for answer choices to eliminate. You will definitely want to read those carefully, practice them, and figure out which ones work best for you. Here though, we're going to address a mindset rather than a particular strategy.

Your odds of guessing an answer correctly depend on how many options you are choosing from.

Number of options left	5	4	3	2	1
Odds of guessing correctly	20%	25%	33%	50%	100%

You can see from this chart just how valuable it is to be able to eliminate incorrect answers and make an educated guess, but there are two things that many test takers do that cause them to miss out on the benefits of guessing:

- Accidentally eliminating the correct answer
- Selecting an answer based on an impression

We'll look at the first one here, and the second one in the next section.

To avoid accidentally eliminating the correct answer, we recommend a thought exercise called **the $5 challenge**. In this challenge, you only eliminate an answer choice from contention if you are willing to bet $5 on it being wrong. Why $5? Five dollars is a small but not insignificant amount of money. It's an amount you could afford to lose but wouldn't want to throw away. And while losing $5 once might not hurt too much, doing it twenty times will set you back $100. In the same way, each small decision you make—eliminating a choice here, guessing on a question there—won't by itself impact your score very much, but when you put them all together, they can make a big difference. By holding each answer choice elimination decision to a higher standard, you can reduce the risk of accidentally eliminating the correct answer.

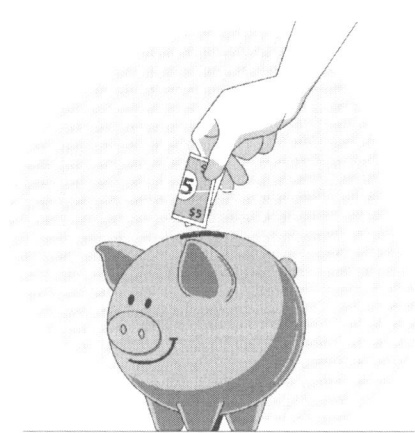

The $5 challenge can also be applied in a positive sense: If you are willing to bet $5 that an answer choice *is* correct, go ahead and mark it as correct.

Summary: Only eliminate an answer choice if you are willing to bet $5 that it is wrong.

Which Answer to Choose

You're taking the test. You've run into a hard question and decided you'll have to guess. You've eliminated all the answer choices you're willing to bet $5 on. Now you have to pick an answer. Why do we even need to talk about this? Why can't you just pick whichever one you feel like when the time comes?

The answer to these questions is that if you don't come into the test with a plan, you'll rely on your impression to select an answer choice, and if you do that, you risk falling into a trap. The test writers know that everyone who takes their test will be guessing on some of the questions, so they intentionally write wrong answer choices to seem plausible. You still have to pick an answer though, and if the wrong answer choices are designed to look right, how can you ever be sure that you're not falling for their trap? The best solution we've found to this dilemma is to take the decision out of your hands entirely. Here is the process we recommend:

Once you've eliminated any choices that you are confident (willing to bet $5) are wrong, select the first remaining choice as your answer.

Whether you choose to select the first remaining choice, the second, or the last, the important thing is that you use some preselected standard. Using this approach guarantees that you will not be enticed into selecting an answer choice that looks right, because you are not basing your decision on how the answer choices look.

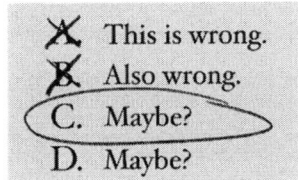

This is not meant to make you question your knowledge. Instead, it is to help you recognize the difference between your knowledge and your impressions. There's a huge difference between thinking an answer is right because of what you know, and thinking an answer is right because it looks or sounds like it should be right.

Summary: To ensure that your selection is appropriately random, make a predetermined selection from among all answer choices you have not eliminated.

Test-Taking Strategies

This section contains a list of test-taking strategies that you may find helpful as you work through the test. By taking what you know and applying logical thought, you can maximize your chances of answering any question correctly!

It is very important to realize that every question is different and every person is different: no single strategy will work on every question, and no single strategy will work for every person. That's why we've included all of them here, so you can try them out and determine which ones work best for different types of questions and which ones work best for you.

Question Strategies

ⓘ READ CAREFULLY

Read the question and the answer choices carefully. Don't miss the question because you misread the terms. You have plenty of time to read each question thoroughly and make sure you understand what is being asked. Yet a happy medium must be attained, so don't waste too much time. You must read carefully and efficiently.

ⓘ CONTEXTUAL CLUES

Look for contextual clues. If the question includes a word you are not familiar with, look at the immediate context for some indication of what the word might mean. Contextual clues can often give you all the information you need to decipher the meaning of an unfamiliar word. Even if you can't determine the meaning, you may be able to narrow down the possibilities enough to make a solid guess at the answer to the question.

ⓘ PREFIXES

If you're having trouble with a word in the question or answer choices, try dissecting it. Take advantage of every clue that the word might include. Prefixes can be a huge help. Usually, they allow you to determine a basic meaning. *Pre-* means before, *post-* means after, *pro-* is positive, *de-* is negative. From prefixes, you can get an idea of the general meaning of the word and try to put it into context.

ⓘ HEDGE WORDS

Watch out for critical hedge words, such as *likely, may, can, often, almost, mostly, usually, generally, rarely,* and *sometimes*. Question writers insert these hedge phrases to cover every possibility. Often an answer choice will be wrong simply because it leaves no room for exception. Be on guard for answer choices that have definitive words such as *exactly* and *always*.

ⓘ SWITCHBACK WORDS

Stay alert for *switchbacks*. These are the words and phrases frequently used to alert you to shifts in thought. The most common switchback words are *but, although,* and *however*. Others include *nevertheless, on the other hand, even though, while, in spite of, despite,* and *regardless of*. Switchback words are important to catch because they can change the direction of the question or an answer choice.

✓ Face Value

When in doubt, use common sense. Accept the situation in the problem at face value. Don't read too much into it. These problems will not require you to make wild assumptions. If you have to go beyond creativity and warp time or space in order to have an answer choice fit the question, then you should move on and consider the other answer choices. These are normal problems rooted in reality. The applicable relationship or explanation may not be readily apparent, but it is there for you to figure out. Use your common sense to interpret anything that isn't clear.

Answer Choice Strategies

✓ Answer Selection

The most thorough way to pick an answer choice is to identify and eliminate wrong answers until only one is left, then confirm it is the correct answer. Sometimes an answer choice may immediately seem right, but be careful. The test writers will usually put more than one reasonable answer choice on each question, so take a second to read all of them and make sure that the other choices are not equally obvious. As long as you have time left, it is better to read every answer choice than to pick the first one that looks right without checking the others.

✓ Answer Choice Families

An answer choice family consists of two (in rare cases, three) answer choices that are very similar in construction and cannot all be true at the same time. If you see two answer choices that are direct opposites or parallels, one of them is usually the correct answer. For instance, if one answer choice says that quantity *x* increases and another either says that quantity *x* decreases (opposite) or says that quantity *y* increases (parallel), then those answer choices would fall into the same family. An answer choice that doesn't match the construction of the answer choice family is more likely to be incorrect. Most questions will not have answer choice families, but when they do appear, you should be prepared to recognize them.

✓ Eliminate Answers

Eliminate answer choices as soon as you realize they are wrong, but make sure you consider all possibilities. If you are eliminating answer choices and realize that the last one you are left with is also wrong, don't panic. Start over and consider each choice again. There may be something you missed the first time that you will realize on the second pass.

✓ Avoid Fact Traps

Don't be distracted by an answer choice that is factually true but doesn't answer the question. You are looking for the choice that answers the question. Stay focused on what the question is asking for so you don't accidentally pick an answer that is true but incorrect. Always go back to the question and make sure the answer choice you've selected actually answers the question and is not merely a true statement.

✓ Extreme Statements

In general, you should avoid answers that put forth extreme actions as standard practice or proclaim controversial ideas as established fact. An answer choice that states the "process should be used in certain situations, if..." is much more likely to be correct than one that states the "process should be discontinued completely." The first is a calm rational statement and doesn't even make a definitive, uncompromising stance, using a hedge word *if* to provide wiggle room, whereas the second choice is far more extreme.

⊘ BENCHMARK

As you read through the answer choices and you come across one that seems to answer the question well, mentally select that answer choice. This is not your final answer, but it's the one that will help you evaluate the other answer choices. The one that you selected is your benchmark or standard for judging each of the other answer choices. Every other answer choice must be compared to your benchmark. That choice is correct until proven otherwise by another answer choice beating it. If you find a better answer, then that one becomes your new benchmark. Once you've decided that no other choice answers the question as well as your benchmark, you have your final answer.

⊘ PREDICT THE ANSWER

Before you even start looking at the answer choices, it is often best to try to predict the answer. When you come up with the answer on your own, it is easier to avoid distractions and traps because you will know exactly what to look for. The right answer choice is unlikely to be word-for-word what you came up with, but it should be a close match. Even if you are confident that you have the right answer, you should still take the time to read each option before moving on.

General Strategies

⊘ TOUGH QUESTIONS

If you are stumped on a problem or it appears too hard or too difficult, don't waste time. Move on! Remember though, if you can quickly check for obviously incorrect answer choices, your chances of guessing correctly are greatly improved. Before you completely give up, at least try to knock out a couple of possible answers. Eliminate what you can and then guess at the remaining answer choices before moving on.

⊘ CHECK YOUR WORK

Since you will probably not know every term listed and the answer to every question, it is important that you get credit for the ones that you do know. Don't miss any questions through careless mistakes. If at all possible, try to take a second to look back over your answer selection and make sure you've selected the correct answer choice and haven't made a costly careless mistake (such as marking an answer choice that you didn't mean to mark). This quick double check should more than pay for itself in caught mistakes for the time it costs.

⊘ PACE YOURSELF

It's easy to be overwhelmed when you're looking at a page full of questions; your mind is confused and full of random thoughts, and the clock is ticking down faster than you would like. Calm down and maintain the pace that you have set for yourself. Especially as you get down to the last few minutes of the test, don't let the small numbers on the clock make you panic. As long as you are on track by monitoring your pace, you are guaranteed to have time for each question.

⊘ DON'T RUSH

It is very easy to make errors when you are in a hurry. Maintaining a fast pace in answering questions is pointless if it makes you miss questions that you would have gotten right otherwise. Test writers like to include distracting information and wrong answers that seem right. Taking a little extra time to avoid careless mistakes can make all the difference in your test score. Find a pace that allows you to be confident in the answers that you select.

⊘ Keep Moving

Panicking will not help you pass the test, so do your best to stay calm and keep moving. Taking deep breaths and going through the answer elimination steps you practiced can help to break through a stress barrier and keep your pace.

Final Notes

The combination of a solid foundation of content knowledge and the confidence that comes from practicing your plan for applying that knowledge is the key to maximizing your performance on test day. As your foundation of content knowledge is built up and strengthened, you'll find that the strategies included in this chapter become more and more effective in helping you quickly sift through the distractions and traps of the test to isolate the correct answer.

Now that you're preparing to move forward into the test content chapters of this book, be sure to keep your goal in mind. As you read, think about how you will be able to apply this information on the test. If you've already seen sample questions for the test and you have an idea of the question format and style, try to come up with questions of your own that you can answer based on what you're reading. This will give you valuable practice applying your knowledge in the same ways you can expect to on test day.

Good luck and good studying!

Five-Week CPHQ Study Plan

On the next few pages, we've provided an optional study plan to help you use this study guide to its fullest potential over the course of five weeks. If you have ten weeks available and want to spread it out more, spend two weeks on each section of the plan.

Below is a quick summary of the subjects covered in each week of the plan.

- Week 1: Quality Leadership and Integration & Quality Review and Accountability
- Week 2: Performance and Process Improvement
- Week 3: Population Health and Care Transitions & Health Data Analytics
- Week 4: Patient Safety & Regulatory and Accreditation
- Week 5: Practice Tests

Please note that not all subjects will take the same amount of time to work through.

Four full-length practice tests are included with this study guide. We recommend saving the last two for after you've completed the study plan. Take these practice tests without any reference materials a day or two before the real thing as practice runs to get you in the mode of answering questions at a good pace.

Week 1: Quality Leadership and Integration & Quality Review and Accountability

INSTRUCTIONAL CONTENT

First, read carefully through the Quality Leadership and Integration & Quality Review and Accountability chapters in this book, checking off your progress as you go:

- ❑ Strategic Planning
- ❑ Stakeholder Engagement
- ❑ Standards and Best Practices
- ❑ Evaluating Compliance with Internal and External Requirements
- ❑ Maintaining Confidentiality

As you read, do the following:

- Highlight any sections, terms, or concepts you think are important
- Draw an asterisk (*) next to any areas you are struggling with
- Watch the review videos to gain more understanding of a particular topic
- Take notes in your notebook or in the margins of this book

After you've read through everything, go back and review any sections that you highlighted or that you drew an asterisk next to, referencing your notes along the way.

Week 2: Performance and Process Improvement

INSTRUCTIONAL CONTENT

First, read carefully through the Performance and Process Improvement chapter in this book, checking off your progress as you go:

- ❏ Quality Improvement Training
- ❏ Communication
- ❏ Teams
- ❏ Evidence-Based Practice
- ❏ Leading and Facilitating Change
- ❏ Performance Improvement Methods
- ❏ Quality Tools and Techniques
- ❏ Monitoring Timeliness
- ❏ Evaluating Effectiveness

As you read, do the following:

- Highlight any sections, terms, or concepts you think are important
- Draw an asterisk (*) next to any areas you are struggling with
- Watch the review videos to gain more understanding of a particular topic
- Take notes in your notebook or in the margins of this book

After you've read through everything, go back and review any sections that you highlighted or that you drew an asterisk next to, referencing your notes along the way.

Week 3: Population Health and Care Transitions & Health Data Analytics

INSTRUCTIONAL CONTENT

First, read carefully through the Population Health and Care Transitions & Health Data Analytics chapters in this book, checking off your progress as you go:

- ❏ Population Health
- ❏ Care Transitions
- ❏ Data Management Systems
- ❏ Measurement and Analysis

As you read, do the following:

- Highlight any sections, terms, or concepts you think are important
- Draw an asterisk (*) next to any areas you are struggling with
- Watch the review videos to gain more understanding of a particular topic
- Take notes in your notebook or in the margins of this book

After you've read through everything, go back and review any sections that you highlighted or that you drew an asterisk next to, referencing your notes along the way.

Week 4: Patient Safety & Regulatory and Accreditation

INSTRUCTIONAL CONTENT

First, read carefully through the Patient Safety & Regulatory and Accreditation chapters in this book, checking off your progress as you go:

- ❏ Patient Rights and Patient Advocacy
- ❏ Technology Solutions to Enhance Patient Safety
- ❏ Enhancing the Culture of Patient Safety
- ❏ Safety Concepts
- ❏ Safety Principles
- ❏ Safety Reviews
- ❏ Accreditation, Certification, and Recognition Options
- ❏ Evaluating Compliance
- ❏ Survey Readiness

As you read, do the following:

- Highlight any sections, terms, or concepts you think are important
- Draw an asterisk (*) next to any areas you are struggling with
- Watch the review videos to gain more understanding of a particular topic
- Take notes in your notebook or in the margins of this book

After you've read through everything, go back and review any sections that you highlighted or that you drew an asterisk next to, referencing your notes along the way.

Week 5: Practice Tests

Your success on test day depends not only on how many hours you put into preparing, but also on whether you prepared the right way. It's good to check along the way to see if your studying is paying off. One of the most effective ways to do this is by taking practice tests to evaluate your progress. Practice tests are useful because they show exactly where you need to improve. Every time you take a practice test, pay special attention to these three groups of questions:

- The questions you got wrong
- The questions you had to guess on, even if you guessed right
- The questions you found difficult or slow to work through

This will show you exactly what your weak areas are, and where you need to devote more study time. Ask yourself why each of these questions gave you trouble. Was it because you didn't understand the material? Was it because you didn't remember the vocabulary? Do you need more repetitions on this type of question to build speed and confidence? Dig into those questions and figure out how you can strengthen your weak areas as you go back to review the material.

PRACTICE TEST #1

Now that you've read over the instructional content, it's time to take a practice test. Complete Practice Test #1. Take this test with **no time constraints**, and feel free to reference the applicable sections of this guide as you go. Once you've finished, check your answers against the provided answer key. For any questions you answered incorrectly, review the answer rationale, and then **go back and review** the applicable sections of the book. The goal in this stage is to understand why you answered the question incorrectly, and make sure that the next time you see a similar question, you will get it right.

PRACTICE TEST #2

Next, complete Practice Test #2. This time, give yourself **3 hours** to complete all of the questions. You should again feel free to reference the guide and your notes, but be mindful of the clock. If you run out of time before you finish all of the questions, mark where you were when time expired, but go ahead and finish taking the practice test. Once you've finished, check your answers against the provided answer key, and as before, review the answer rationale for any that you answered incorrectly and then go back and review the associated instructional content. Your goal is still to increase understanding of the content but also to get used to the time constraints you will face on the test.

As you go along, keep in mind that the practice test is just that: practice. Memorizing these questions and answers will not be very helpful on the actual test because it is unlikely to have any of the same exact questions. If you only know the right answers to the sample questions, you won't be prepared for the real thing. **Study the concepts** until you understand them fully, and then you'll be able to answer any question that shows up on the test.

Quality Leadership and Integration

Strategic Planning

CERTIFIED PROFESSIONAL IN HEALTHCARE QUALITY

The Certified Professional in Healthcare Quality (CPHQ) has a unique and broad responsibility in an organization. The CPHQ promotes and supports quality assurance, safety, and effective healthcare. The quality professional must also have the expertise to design, implement, and evaluate **process improvement activities**. The CPHQ must:

- Develop data collection and measurement procedures in order to evaluate outcomes
- Provide education for administration and staff
- Coordinate activities related to licensure, accreditation, standards, and regulations
- Provide leadership as an agent of change within the organization
- Identify organizational needs and opportunities for improvement
- Prepare organization-wide plans, including quality management, patient safety, utilization, and risk management
- Document activities and provide summary reports to leadership and the governing board
- Facilitate interdisciplinary participation and teams
- Differentiate among a variety of organizational needs

TIME MANAGEMENT TECHNIQUES

Time management is an important function of leaders who must not only manage their own time, but must also model time management and schedule others' time effectively. Steps for effective time management are:

1. Plan	Create goals. Establish schedules for yearly, monthly, and daily activities. Plan each day in advance.
2. Create a task list	Update the task list daily, including routine tasks, so that all can be completed.
3. Prioritize	Rank the order in which tasks are to be accomplished, beginning with high priority items.
4. Minimize paper handling	Handle a paper or task once, instead of shuffling it about and dealing with it repeatedly.
5. Use time effectively	Avoid wasted time by starting meetings on schedule, and ask a timekeeper to monitor the time and announce when the time is up. Work efficiently, paying attention to necessary details.
6. Delegate	Determine which tasks can be delegated to others and do not micromanage those tasks.
7. Use computer technology	Avoid paper when possible. Keep calendars and lists on the computer for easy updating. Utilize email and the internet.
8. Avoid procrastination	Address needs when they are realized rather than waiting until the situation becomes urgent.

ORGANIZATION-WIDE STRATEGIC PLANNING

Organization-wide strategic planning requires that an organization examine its needs, community, and customers and establish goals for the **near future** (2–4 years) and the **extended future** (10–15 years). Strategic planning must be based on assessments, both internal and external, to determine the present courses of action, needed changes, priorities, and methodologies to effect change. The focus of strategic planning must be on the development of services. The organization identifies customer needs, develops services, and then markets those services.

Organization-wide strategic planning includes the following:

- Collect data and conduct an external analysis of customer needs in relation to regulations and demographics
- Analyze internal services and functions
- Identify and understand key issues, including the strengths and weaknesses of the organization, potential opportunities, and negative impacts
- Develop revised mission and vision statements that identify core values
- Establish specific goals and objectives, based on findings

CUSTOMER NEEDS AND SATISFACTION

In any healthcare organization, it is critical to thoroughly understand the needs of customers in order to provide satisfactory outcomes. While identifying customer needs and satisfaction can be challenging, there are strategic ways to approach the assessment of customer needs and satisfaction to ensure that these concepts are integrated into the organization's strategic plan.

First, one must have a clear understanding of who one's customers are and how to categorize them to best assess satisfaction. In general, a **customer** is the recipient of a product or service. More specifically, customers can be categorized as either external or internal.

Within healthcare, patients are considered **external customers**. Patients want to avoid complications and regain their health without worrying about a plan. The **internal customers** include:

- **Hospital administrators**, who want a cost-effective plan, increased productivity, and reduced liability
- **Physicians**, who want to provide positive outcomes for patients, and assistance in providing care
- **Nurses** who want a practical, efficient plan that can be implemented without increasing their workload
- **Environmental services workers**, who want a plan that relates to the resources available in each department
- **Accreditation agencies**, who want a plan that provides documented proof of the organization's compliance with accreditation standards
- **Communities/community agencies**, who want a plan that meets the needs of the various populations they represent
- **Insurance companies**, who want a cost-saving plan
- **Suppliers**, who want a profitable, efficient plan

Secondly, one must consider the **voice of the customer (VOC)**. Voice of the customer is a term used to describe the process of capturing information from consumers regarding their experience with a product or service and using that data to determine customer requirements.

The process of determining the voice of the customer is comprised of 4 components:

- **Customer needs** are the benefit of receiving the product or service, as described by the customer. This is typically communicated through qualitative interviews with customers to identify the experience of the product or service from a customer perspective and adjust accordingly.
- **Hierarchical structure** categorizes customer needs into primary, secondary, or tertiary needs. Primary needs are those communicated by the customer that need to be built into the strategic plan. Secondary needs indicate specific actions that must take place to then satisfy the primary needs and overall strategy. Tertiary needs are operational details to allow for the entire plan to come together.
- **Priorities** for customers can differ. It is important to have a clear understanding of which aspects of a product or service hold higher priority for a customer.
- **Customer perceptions of performance** help organizations understand if there are gaps in the delivered product or service from a customer perspective.

ORGANIZATIONAL ETHICS

Organizational ethics is the value system at work within an organization. While almost all healthcare organizations have a written code of ethics, an ethical organization embodies that code within all processes, including:

- A code of right conduct governing staff relationships with patients and the public
- Recognition of the patient's right to quality care and respect for personal religious beliefs, culture, and psychosocial values
- Transparency in disclosure of information and accountability
- Adherence to regulations and best practices
- Recognition of the need to empower staff and patients
- Leadership without intimidation or fear tactics
- Standard, open guidelines for organ donation, procurement, and research projects
- Maintenance of a bioethics committee to provide guidance related to ethical issues in healthcare

DEVELOPING AN ORGANIZATIONAL VISION STATEMENT

An organizational vision statement requires the CPHQ to analyze both internal and external customer-supplier relationships, so a statement about what the organization intends to become can be created. The vision statement is the commitment that the organization is making to its stakeholders. The vision statement outlines future goals, rather than focusing on what has already been achieved. Make the vision statement in one sentence or a short paragraph, for example:

> *Hospital X will be the leader in providing sustainable quality patient-centered care to (name the community), and to improve the physical and mental health of community members.*

Follow the vision statement with an explanation of terms, so that such concepts as "sustainable" and "patient-centered" are clarified for the reader. For example, if "sustainable" is part of the vision statement, then the explanation should include "the need to function within budget constraints, while providing optimum care."

Developing an Organizational Mission Statement

The mission statement of an organization reflects the current status of the organization and describes, in broad terms, the purpose of the organization and its role in the community. Develop the mission statement in response to data and program analysis, and with input from all members of the organization. The mission statement identifies the organization or program, states its function, and outlines the purpose and strategy of the program, for example:

> *Hospital X is a collaborative group of professionals, physicians, administrators, nurses, and support staff. The mission of Hospital X is to promote the health and safety of its patients, visitors, and staff, and to provide outstanding quality health care services to (name the community).*

The mission statement should in some way include a commitment to quality and patient care, and the need to serve the community. In many cases, the mission statement is followed by detailed explanations, which may include statements of organizational values, philosophy, and history.

Developing Goals and Objectives

Goals and objectives support the mission and vision statements, so complete them at the same time to determine if the mission and vision statements can be realized, and explain how that will happen.

Goals should be achievable aims, essentially end results, developed for specific units of the organization or the organization in general, focusing on improving performance. Best practice is to ensure that goals are SMART:

- **S**pecific
- **M**easurable
- **A**chievable
- **R**elevant
- **T**ime-bound

An example of a SMART goal is:

> *The Neonatal Intensive Care Unit will reduce surgical site infections by 30% from 2020 levels by the end of the calendar year by monitoring staff adherence to disinfection protocol prior to surgery.*

In healthcare quality management, the goals must be based on knowledge about functions and processes within the organization, and prioritized accordingly, as part of achieving positive patient outcomes.

Objectives are the measurable steps taken to achieve goals and should concretely describe who will be doing what, when and how. In the case of infections, an objective might include:

> *An Infection Control practitioner will audit antibiotic use, and the Physicians' Internal Medicine Committee will establish an antibiotic prophylaxis protocol within 6 months.*

Objectives must be measurable, include a timeline, and identify who is responsible for achieving the objective.

STEPS FOR DEVELOPING AN ACTION PLAN

Developing an action plan requires the following steps:

1. Monitor and assess the problems for a period of one month, if possible.
2. Prioritize the problems.
3. Assign teams to focus on particular problems, based on their knowledge of or participation in the process selected, and their commitment to improvement.
4. Coach each team to write a performance improvement action plan.
5. Systematically identify reasons for variation in a process. Perform a root cause analysis. Identify feasible changes in process.
6. Formulate an action plan that clearly outlines the expected outcomes, steps in the plan, responsibility, timeline, and types of measurements to use for monitoring and evaluation.
7. Conduct a pilot test, after determining the timeframe, sample size, and locations.
8. Analyze data from the pilot test.
9. Modify the action plan, and conduct further pilot testing.
10. Commit resources to the action plan. Involve individuals, departments, and areas involved in the process, and the appropriate leaders.
11. Implement the action plan on a limited trial basis, after providing training and rescheduling staff.
12. Determine the most effective performance measures.
13. Establish a timeline for full implementation.
14. Evaluate the trial implementation and make changes or conduct further analysis, as indicated.
15. Provide clear, detailed communication to all those involved in the process.
16. Incorporate action plans into organizational procedures, and fully implement the action plan.
17. Continue to monitor implementation through performance measures, data collection, surveys, and other feedback from those involved.
18. Monitor and evaluate the impact on patient care, and whether the goals were achieved through changes in process.
19. Document the implementation process and the results.
20. Disseminate the report organization-wide.

ANALYSIS OF PROCESSES IN CURRENT USE

The analysis of processes currently in use is a critical step in the development of action plans for performance improvement. It involves the aggregation of data (gathering it together) and analysis of each part of the data. The data is used to facilitate change only, not for disciplinary reasons. The purpose of the analysis process is to develop a clear profile of the organization's current level of performance, the stability of current processes, areas of needed improvement, strategies for improving processes, and consistency of design and priorities. The goals of process analysis are:

- **Internal comparison**, which reviews patterns and trends, sentinel events, and upper and lower control limits (guardrails).
- **External comparison** as a reference base of the manner in which others perform similar processes and their outcomes.
- **Standards comparison**, which compares internal data with knowledge-based practice guidelines and regulations.
- **Benchmark comparison**, which may be internal or external, and compares data with benchmark or best practice data.

LINKING PATIENT SAFETY ACTIVITIES WITH STRATEGIC GOALS

Linking patient safety activities with the strategic goals of the organization is an important step in developing a plan for patient safety. The governing board and leadership must re-evaluate the strategic goals periodically, and revise them as part of the organization's commitment to safety. Strategic goals may be expressed in terms that are very broad, such as "improve patient safety," but these broad goals should be coupled with more specific objectives, such as "decrease post-operative infections." As part of the linkage procedure, activities must be identified that relate to each strategic goal and objective, and the data collection method and expected measurable outcomes should be specified for each activity, with a timeline. For example, "decrease the number of surgical site infections by 40% by September 1, 2021." Goals for measurable outcomes should be based on assessment and data, so that they are achievable with adherence to performance improvement activities.

PRIORITIZING PROCESS IMPROVEMENT ACTIVITIES

Many activities will be identified for process improvement. It is unfeasible to deal with all of them simultaneously, so the CPHQ must **prioritize** them for sequential investigation. Defer or ignore single events or those with low impact by determining which hold the most value.

$$Value = \frac{Quality\ of\ Service + Outcome}{Cost}$$

Assemble teams that include upper management and subject matter experts (SME) who are familiar with the needs of the organization. The team decides on which processes they should focus and sets the performance measures.

The team considers which issues require more analysis and looks at existing outcomes that need improvement:

- Risk management and safety violations if the problem is not resolved
- Probability of improved outcomes
- Overall impact on efficiency and delivery of care
- Number of parties involved
- Costs in staff, time, and money

- Relation to mission, vision, and strategic goals
- Frequency and duration of the problem

PRIORITIZATION MATRIX

A prioritization matrix determines which item takes precedence, based on pre-selected criteria. The steps for forming a prioritization matrix are:

- Brainstorm to generate a list of problems or options.
- List selection criteria, e.g., cost, patient outcome, and safety.
- Determine the relative value of each criterion and assign weighted points accordingly. For example, each vote for safety is worth 3 points, patient outcome is worth 2 points, and cost is worth 1 point.
- Create a table with enough columns to fit the number of criteria.
- Title the left column "Problems/Options." Title the middle column "Criteria". Title the right column "Total Points."

Team members vote by one of these methods:

- Check-marking those criteria that apply
- Using a scale from 1–5, where 1 is the least important and 5 is the most important
- Using a yes/no or + and - system

The scores are then totaled to rank the priorities.

MULTI-VOTING

Multi-voting is a procedure to prioritize and reach consensus when selecting process improvement activities:

- Review the initial list for redundancies and similarities. Combine like items if the group agrees. Restate the item as agreed by the team.
- Number the remaining items on the list, without prioritizing them.
- Select a voting method, such as colored dots, a point system, or a ranking system. A simple method is one-half plus one (one dot more than half the number of items).
- Vote using the chosen method and tally the votes to determine which items have the most votes.
- Discuss the items that received the most votes.
- Eliminate items with no votes or few votes.
- Repeat the voting and discussion procedure until the list has narrowed. Use voting to prioritize the remaining items.

AFFINITY DIAGRAM

Use an affinity diagram to brainstorm and organize more than 15 ideas, items, or issues into major categories:

- Brainstorm to generate a list of ideas. Write each one on a Post-it note or 3x5 card.
- Display the Post-its or cards at random on a table or wall.
- Sort the ideas into groups, silently and quickly. Find two ideas that go together. Place them to one side. Add to each group until all cards have been either grouped or stand isolated.

- Discuss each group and agree to a title for each group. If some groups have sub-groups, then create subheadings and move one group under another as a sub-group.
- Draw a diagram with the idea at the top, the titles below, and the subheadings beneath.

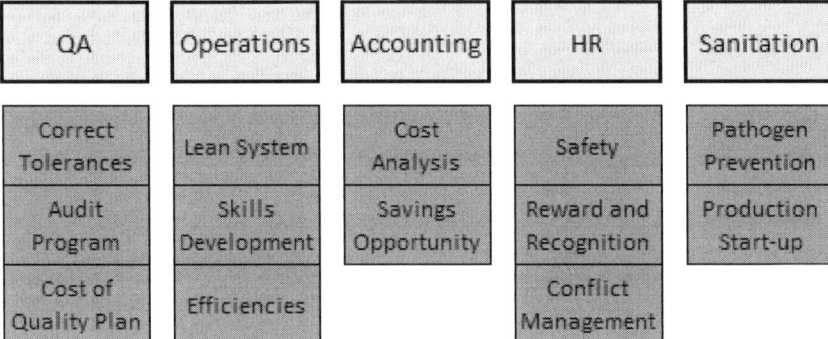

Brainstorming

Brainstorming is a component of almost all planning and prioritizing activities. Brainstorming generates ideas about problems, process, solutions, or other criteria in a short time frame. Brainstorming may be structured, with each person in the group providing an idea in rotation, or unstructured, with participants contributing at will. There are 5 primary steps:

1. Establish the purpose of the brainstorming and a time frame.
2. Decide on a structured or unstructured approach.
3. Allow time for general discussion or individual thought.
4. List ideas according to the approach. Write ideas on a white board, flip chart, overhead projector acetate, or computer, so the group can look at the list.
5. Discuss items, clarify, and combine like items as the group agrees.

Ask members to rate or rank items on the list individually. Assign points to each item. Prioritize the list accordingly.

Checklists and Deployment Charts

Checklists are an effective tool to track progress during a performance improvement initiative and ensure that critical tasks are completed. **Checklists** may be organized in a format that best suits the tasks at hand. For example, an ordered checklist may be best when certain tasks must be completed before others. An itemized checklist is a more thorough checklist format, containing full detail of each task during a project. Healthcare quality professionals must be able to develop and monitor checklists as a project progresses to identify potential barriers early on and adjust as needed to ensure success of the project.

Deployment charts are a performance improvement tool that assists with development of and adherence to the project schedule. Critical tasks are identified to help prioritize work and responsibility is assigned for specific aspects of the project. A deployment chart is typically designed in a grid format with shading that makes it easy to quickly glance at and identify milestones achieved and specific roles within the group.

Governance Infrastructure

Understanding the governance infrastructure of an organization is necessary for integrating quality findings. Organizations incorporated by state charter are required to have a governing body, which carries legal authority and responsibility for all care provided by the organization. The governing body is organized under by-laws, in accordance with both state and federal regulations. The factors that impact the board's ability to effect change are:

- Size and structure of the board
- Experience and knowledge of its members
- Management infrastructure, including leadership, objectives, agendas, meetings, education, and assessment
- Functions, roles, and responsibilities, such as formulating vision and strategic goals, ensuring quality, developing policies, decision-making, and oversight

INTEGRATING QUALITY FINDINGS
INTEGRATING QUALITY FINDINGS INTO GOVERNANCE AND MANAGEMENT ACTIVITIES

Integrating quality findings into governance and management activities requires a commitment from the governing board and administration to restructuring and re-engineering. Findings must be incorporated into the strategic goals, and by-laws and administrative policies must be realigned to reflect a change in focus. This process requires broad changes to offer a seamless continuum of care:

- Aligning payment and incentive systems, to tie rewards to clinical objectives for improving health care
- Establishing a new culture of organization-wide management, rather than focusing management on departments
- Integrating the administrative and management infrastructure to include planning for resource allocation, marketing, human resource development, and quality care
- Assessing populations to determine needs within the community
- Providing services in accordance with needs assessment, including adequate access to services
- Utilizing technology for assessment and evaluation
- Establishing critical care pathways and protocols, and utilizing continuous improvement processes with interdisciplinary teams
- Establishing case management

INTEGRATING QUALITY FINDINGS IN BY-LAWS

The by-laws of the governing body define lines of authority, responsibility, accountability and communication within the organization. By-laws specify the formation and structure of the governing board, and the procedures for selecting officers and committees. The by-laws establish the relationship between the governing board and the medical staff and define conflicts of interest. By-laws specify lines of authority and responsibility at all levels in the organization related to quality, safety, patient care, credentialing, privileging, and performance improvement. Budget development and approval of the budget are central responsibilities of the governing board because budget considerations directly impact quality of patient care and the ability of the organization to carry out substantial changes. As part of the budget process, the by-laws provide that the governing board plans for organization-wide services.

INTEGRATING QUALITY FINDINGS INTO STRATEGIC GOALS

The governing board must establish a method by which quality management activities and issues are reported to them. Once the board has established **strategic goals** based on quality findings and input from quality professionals, the board must ensure integration of the findings into governance and management. It must:

- Provide organization-wide support for strategic goals
- Utilize performance improvement measures as part of business planning and resource allocation
- Support the use of performance measures to provide current information about performance organization-wide, such as with balanced scorecards or dashboards
- Provide resources for education and training
- Participate in oversight activities through the creation of oversight teams or committees, including review of summary reports regarding performance improvement activities, public reporting, and validation of compliance with licensing, credentialing, and privileging regulations or by-laws

INTEGRATING QUALITY FINDINGS INTO MANAGEMENT ROLES

Management has a critical role in integrating quality findings into their activities. Managers must consistently look toward the future of an organization, govern growth, work toward restructuring and internalizing change, manage knowledge, and integrate best practices into processes to ensure quality. Managers must:

- Exhibit a commitment to performance improvement and create a culture of quality
- Empower staff to facilitate change
- Provide adequate training, support, and resources for performance improvement activities
- Participate in the quality improvement process and incorporate it into job descriptions
- Evaluate compliance with quality performance goals
- Monitor effectiveness of performance activities and conduct evaluations
- Provide continuous education regarding quality performance to all levels of the organization
- Provide reports and education to the governing board

LEADERSHIP

TYPES OF LEADERS

The four types of leaders are:

Charismatic	The charismatic leader depends on personal charm to influence people and is very persuasive. However, charismatic leaders have limited effectiveness because they make followers of employees, and relate to one group, rather than the organization as a whole.
Bureaucratic	The bureaucrat follows the organization's rules exactly and expects everyone else to do the same. Bureaucrats are most effective in handling cash flow or managing work in dangerous work environments. Bureaucrats may engender respect but are not conducive to change or creativity.
Autocratic	The autocrat makes decisions independently, and strictly enforces rules. Team members often feel left out of the decision-making process and may not be supportive. Autocratic leaders are most effective in crisis situations but may have difficulty with staff commitment for routine work.
Consultative	The consultant presents a decision to staff and welcomes their input and questions, although the original decision rarely changes. Consultative leadership is most effective when gaining the support of staff is critical to the success of proposed changes.

LEADERSHIP STYLES

The seven leadership styles are:

Participatory	A participatory style means the leader presents a potential decision and then makes the final decision based on input from individual employees or teams. Participatory leadership is time-consuming and may result in compromises that are not wholly satisfactory to either management or staff, but participation motivates employees, who feel their expertise is valued.
Democratic	A democratic style means the leader presents a problem and asks individual employees or teams to arrive at a solution, although the leader usually makes the final decision. Democratic leadership may delay decision-making, but employees and teams are often more committed to the solutions because of their input.
Empowering	An empowering style means the leader shares power with employees, allowing them to engage in decision making and encouraging their input in all aspects of the business. This leadership style motivates the team and ensures that all employees have the necessary resources to be successful in their role.
Transactional	A transactional style means that the leader views the dynamic of leadership as an exchange based on rewards and punishment. For example, by meeting specific goals, team members are rewarded, creating positive reinforcement. Transactional leaders use this perspective to motivate employees and create structure within the organization.
Transformational	A transformational style means that the leader inspires and motivates employees to work towards a common goal. This leadership style encourages team members to perform above and beyond the status quo, increasing intrinsic motivation.
Situational	A situational style means that a leader adapts their style based on the needs of the team and organization. Situational leadership encompasses six different styles: coaching, pacesetting, democratic, affiliative, authoritative and coercive.
Laissez-faire (free rein)	A laissez-faire style means the leader exerts indirect control, allowing employees/teams to make decisions independently, with little interference. Laissez-faire may be effective leadership if the teams are highly skilled and strongly motivated, but in many cases laissez-faire leadership is the product of poor management skills and little is accomplished because of lack of direction.

PROFESSIONAL LEADERSHIP AND ACCOUNTABILITY FOR NURSING'S ROLE

Nurses, especially those in leadership positions, have a responsibility to assist others with **professional leadership and accountability** within the healthcare team and community. Collaboration requires an ongoing commitment that includes mentoring, coaching, and teaching others. Nursing must be involved in the following:

- Making decisions at all levels of an organization/facility
- Taking an active role in strategic planning
- Assuming responsibility for standards of nursing care
- Assessing and selecting equipment, supplies, and electronic information systems

- Assisting with planning for utilization of resources
- Analyzing all decisions with respect to patient outcomes
- Supporting staff education and development, including training for management positions, and offering opportunities to acquire continuing education hours
- Facilitating access to research and both internal and external resources
- Allowing staff members time to consider their place in the organization and in their own practices

CREATING STAFF COMMITMENT

Leadership must be consistent and succeeds by providing staff with direction and guidance that shows by example, explaining why things need to be done, rather than directing how this must be achieved. A good leader fosters values by focusing on the right way to do things, rather than on errors or poor performance. By engaging staff in all parts of the process, a leader engenders a sense of **commitment in the staff**. Commitment cannot be achieved through rules, regulations, threats, and criticism. A good leader must demonstrate integrity, welcome diversity, be open-minded, and search for competence. While a leader must have a thorough understanding of the organization/facility and its work, he or she must be able to perceive holistically. The leader must motivate others by providing structure, order, and sound decision-making. The leader must both learn and teach in order to create positive change.

Stakeholder Engagement

ENGAGING STAKEHOLDERS TO PROMOTE QUALITY AND SAFETY

PROMOTING QUALITY AND SAFETY THROUGH DISASTER/EMERGENCY PREPAREDNESS PLANS

Disaster/emergency preparedness plans should be in place based on the Hospital Incident Command System (HICS) (formerly the Hospital Emergency Incident Command System [HEICS]), which provides a model for management, responsibilities, and communication. Key stakeholders include the CPHQ, the disaster response team, the administration, the public health department, police, first responders, and fire departments. Disasters can include a multi-casualty influx of individuals from a community emergency, such as a train accident; an epidemic; a fire or other internal hospital problem requiring evacuation; or inadequate staffing to safely treat ED individuals.

Plans should include/address the following:

- Readily available information and disaster preparedness drills
- Activation of the plan, including the individual(s) responsible
- Chain of command
- Facility damage assessment, usually conducted by the plant safety officer
- Hospital/ED capacity to receive individuals
- Triage, including in the community and in the ED
- Transfer protocols for distributing individuals to other facilities
- Staffing, including a telephone tree to notify staff to report to the facility
- Intra- and inter-facility communication and communication with pre-hospital EMS personnel
- Supplies on hand and methods to obtain added supplies
- Delineation of receiving and treatment areas

PROMOTING QUALITY AND SAFETY THROUGH CORPORATE COMPLIANCE

The Office of Inspector General of HHS issues **corporate compliance** guidance for different types of healthcare organizations. Corporate compliance requires adherence to state and federal regulations and legal and ethical standards. Because compliance issues are so broad and complex, the organization should have a compliance officer with expertise to review all compliance issues and ensure that the organization complies. Compliance issues include the following:

- Privacy and security concerns of HIPAA, HITECH, including conducting audit trails
- Accountability standards: Discipline, confidentiality, and privacy policies
- Regulatory requirements: Include ADA, CMS, CLIA, EMTALA, OSHA, EEOC, Anti-Kickback Statute, Stark Law (limiting referrals by physicians), Fair Labor Standards Act, Family and Medical Leave Act, and Federal Wage Garnishment Law
- Record retention policies and practices
- Screening/Employment standards and practices, including appropriate interviewing (hiring and exit)
- Third party due diligence: Vendors, contractual agreements
- Communication of regulatory requirements and education in compliance issues
- Risk assessment and compliance audits (internal, external)
- Investigations and disclosures of non-compliance

- Government sanctions lists: Including country-specific lists as well as terrorism and narcotics sanctions lists, and OIG exclusions of individuals
- Organizational transparency and culture of compliance

Promoting Quality and Safety Through Provider Networks

Provider networks are specific types of healthcare insurance plans in which claims from healthcare providers in a network are reimbursed at a higher level than claims from healthcare providers who are outside of the network. The provider network comprises a group of healthcare providers (physicians, therapists, advanced practice registered nurses [APRNs], hospitals) who have a contractual agreement to provide services at a prescribed fee via a paid-provider organization (PPO), a health maintenance organization (HMO) or an exclusive provider organization (EPO):

- In a **PPO**, patients are not required to select a primary care provider or to obtain a referral to see other in-network providers. With these plans, patients are responsible for an annual deductible and copay; however, they must pay additional fees for seeing providers outside of this network.
- In an **HMO**, patients must receive all care from their in-network provider. They are required to identify a PCP who is responsible for coordination of care and referring to outside specialists as deemed clinically necessary.
- In an **EPO**, patients must receive care exclusively from providers within this network. Services are limited to preventive or medically necessary care.

The board of directors and administration are often key stakeholders in utilizing a provider network rather than other types of plans because provider networks provide negotiated discounts for treatment and may also provide substantial savings in healthcare costs. However, costs may also be substantial for participants who choose an out-of-network provider, and individuals seeking care must first determine which healthcare providers are in the network. Provider networks often have preauthorization requirements, such as before expensive diagnostic procedures (MRI, angiography) or surgeries.

Focus Groups

Focus groups are valuable tools for assessing customer needs. Choose 8–12 participants who share characteristics with the group that needs to be researched (e.g., age, ethnic background, community affiliation, health history, healthcare providers). Arrange for the group to meet for 1.5–2 hours for a focused discussion on a particular topic. Identify a facilitator or moderator and a recorder. It may be beneficial to observe from behind a one-way mirror, such as the kind found in police interrogation rooms. Non-traditional focus groups are sometimes conducted by conference telephone calls, internet groups, or videoconferences. Focus groups are told the topic before the discussion, and often begin by sharing stories. For example, if emergency care is the focus, then all participants share their experiences in an emergency department. Then, the facilitator asks the group to focus on a few aspects of some stories in detail. The stories are retold, and the facilitator asks questions to obtain more details. The facilitator asks the group to respond to the stories with their reactions, comments, and questions. The recorder prepares a transcript of the meeting for study.

Using Traditional Focus Groups to Assess Customer Needs and Expectations

The advantages of using traditional focus groups, rather than electronic groups, to assess customer needs and expectations are:

- The facilitator guides the discussion to ensure that topics of interest are covered adequately, and that all members participate, keeping the discussion focused on the topic.
- The focus can be modified as needed, to allow for discussion of new ideas.
- The non-confrontational method of allowing people to share experiences allows for expression of new ideas.
- Administration or researchers may observe the interactions through the one-way mirror and communicate with the facilitator regarding further questions.
- The participants are fully involved in the process.
- Nonverbal behavior, such as facial expressions and gestures, can be observed.
- Participants are pre-screened and identified prior to the focus group meeting, and participants are not influenced by others outside the group, as may occur with telephone or internet focus groups.

Strategic Quality Planning to Promote Performance Improvement

Strategic quality planning to promote performance improvement must begin at the top level of management, with a commitment to facilitate change at all levels, and to provide the financial resources that make these changes possible. Every strategic quality plan begins with a clear definition of quality as it applies to customers, and relates this to the organization's mission and vision statements, goals, and objectives. Processes are redesigned to achieve quality. Organizational performance measurements are modified to ensure regulatory compliance. **Total quality management** (TQM) is at the center of all planning. An organization-wide model for quality performance must be used that includes at least the following:

- Assessment
- Planning
- Implementation
- Evaluation of continuous improvement

The planning process must be documented and must contain an action plan that ensures ongoing evaluation of progress.

Interdisciplinary Collaboration

Interdisciplinary collaboration is absolutely critical to medical practice if the needs and best interests of the patients and families are central. Interdisciplinary practice begins with the nurse and physician, and extends to pharmacists, social workers, occupational therapists, physiotherapists, nutritionists, lab technologists, and a wide range of allied healthcare providers, all of whom cooperate in diagnosis and treatment. State regulations determine how much autonomy a nurse has in diagnosing, treating, and prescribing. While nurses have gained more legal rights, they have also become more dependent on collaboration with others for their expertise and for referrals, if the patient's needs extend beyond the nurse's ability to provide assistance. Some states require direct supervision of nurses by physicians, dentists, or other licensed practitioners. Other states allow indirect supervisory arrangements, depending on the circumstances. For example, nurse practitioners have much more latitude than new grads.

Performance and Process Improvement

Quality Improvement Training

PERFORMANCE IMPROVEMENT TRAINING

These steps should be followed when planning organizational performance improvement training:

- Perform a needs assessment and be mindful of the organizational outcomes to be achieved.
- Pretest the staff's current level of knowledge for targeted information.
- Use strategic goals to establish specific learning goals and objectives tied to the mission and vision of the organization.
- Determine methods of outcomes measurement.
- Assess staff learning styles (visual, auditory, kinesthetic) and teaching techniques to develop teaching strategies.
- Develop course materials.
- Train instructors or assistants as necessary.
- Pilot test training materials and the program with a small group and use their feedback to make modifications.
- Implement the revised training program.
- Measure to determine outcomes.

ADDIE MODEL OF ORGANIZATIONAL PERFORMANCE IMPROVEMENT TRAINING

Florida State University developed the **ADDIE Model** for instructional systems development. It provides an outline for development of training programs in five steps:

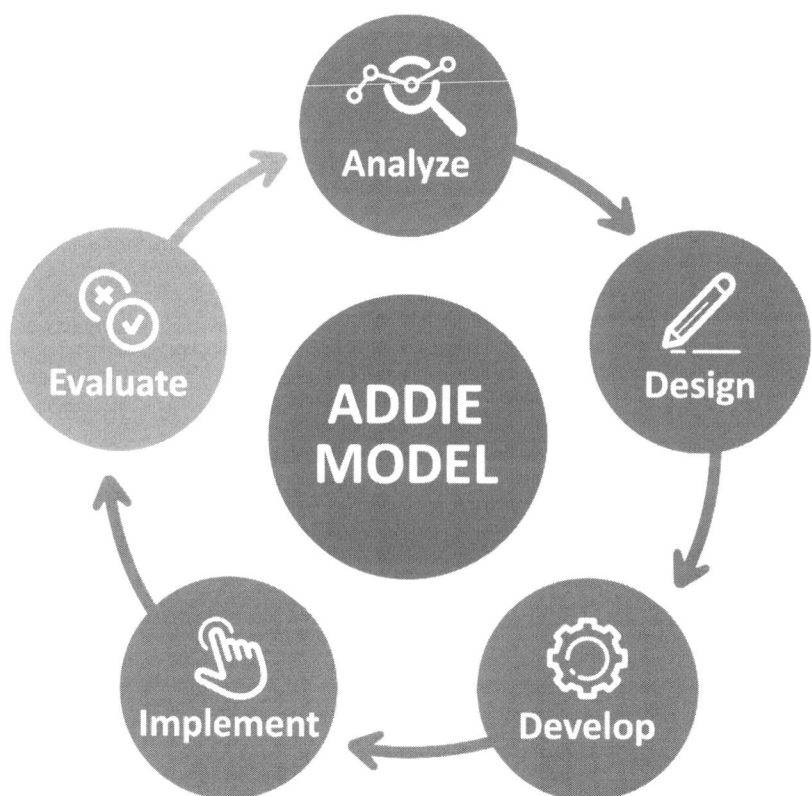

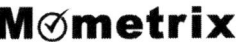

1. Analyze	Assess the needs of the organization, the current level of knowledge, and the specific types of staff training needs, including goals and outcomes. Obtain information about needs from those involved in targeted processes. Identify the training facilities, resources, and any limitations. Develop learning objectives.
2. Design	Plan the training based on what the learners already know and need to know. Clarify the strategy for instruction and course format in a written instructional plan.
3. Develop	Create course materials based on the analysis and design plan. Present the course for review to ensure it is accurate and complete. Pilot the course and review it again.
4. Implement	Provide a training timeline and schedule of courses. Book classrooms and enroll learners. Coordinate with supervisors to ensure staff can attend classes. If extra instructors are needed, train them. Print or purchase course materials. Prepare certificates or participation records. Arrange for A/V equipment, computers, internet access, and travel plans as necessary.
5. Evaluate	Pretest and posttest learners to find if the course material was retained. Distribute a satisfaction survey for immediate feedback about whether learners liked the course and felt it met their expectations and the stated goals. Remember that long-term outcomes related to actual performance improvement are more difficult to quantify and may take months.

FACILITY'S ORIENTATION PROGRAM

The CPHQ's participation in the facility's orientation program signals the administration's commitment to performance improvement. The CPHQ should not design stand-alone orientation classes, but should integrate orientation with other presentations so that the new hires understand how performance improvement is a multidisciplinary focus of the facility. Cover specific procedures, such as hand hygiene and barrier precautions, in detail. Give general information about surveillance and indicators. Staff must understand the processes in place for both patient and staff safety, and what action Human Resources will take if staff does not comply with performance improvement measures. New hires should know what all departments do to focus on process improvement, rather than just their own department.

CULTURAL DIVERSITY, SENSITIVITY, AND AWARENESS
FACILITATING AWARENESS OF DIVERSITY ISSUES AMONG STAFF

Cultural diversity is an integral part of the care plan, so always address it during in-service training. Do not assume all members of an ethnic or cultural group share the same values. Assess the patient's individual variations, and ethnic group. Make basic cultural guidelines available to staff, which outline appropriate:

- Eye contact
- Proximity
- Gestures
- Family dynamics (e.g., in patriarchal Mexican culture, the eldest male speaks for the patient; in Muslim cultures, females resist care by males.)
- Use of traditional healers or cultural medicines that must be incorporated into a care plan
- End-of-life care

Arrange for translators in case of a language barrier to ensure adequate communication. Get an emergency contact list of religious visitors (priests, rabbis, mullahs, etc.) from Chaplaincy. Ensure religious visitors are orientated, have hospital photo IDs, and parking passes. Understand and accept the attitudes and beliefs of the patient in relation to care and treatment, and treat all patients and family members with respect.

TAILORING CARE DELIVERY TO MEET THE DIVERSE NEEDS AND STRENGTHS OF PATIENTS

Diverse patients who are ethnic, cultural, or lifestyle minorities often receive less than optimal care from healthcare workers. The CPHQ ensures all diverse patients and their families receive equal quality care by helping staff deliver care tailored to meet the individual needs of their patients. Begin by asking staff to examine their own attitudes. Hold an open discussion about diversity to help staff gain self-awareness, and determine if their ideas are stereotypical or based on inaccurate knowledge. Format care plans to specifically address diversity issues, so that discussions of diversity and preferences are part of care plan development, and not an addendum. The initial patient assessment should include questions about family, country of birth, educational level, religious preferences, and native language, with explanations about why the questions are asked, to establish a relationship of trust and respect. Encourage the patient and family to express their individual differences.

DEVELOPING CULTURAL DIVERSITY PLANS USING EXPERIENTIAL KNOWLEDGE

Acceptance and responsiveness to diversity requires an organizational commitment with ongoing in-service training to assist staff. The CPHQ can develop the following:

- **Multicultural advisory committees** with community representatives to provide insight and determine areas for research or outreach to diverse groups.
- **Mentors or consultants** who provide guidance to staff dealing with diversity issues.
- **Adaptation** of patient information, surveys, and family materials for diverse groups (e.g., culturally appropriate adaptations, translation into various languages for readers who are not proficient in English, pictorial direction signs).
- **Hiring, retention, and promotion strategies** to build a diverse workforce that is representative of the community it serves.
- **In-service training** on how to work with interpreters.
- **Integrated cultural content** throughout the training curriculum, with specific information about cultural attitudes toward intimacy, sexuality, end-of-life, mental and physical illness, drug use, and general health.
- **Presentations**, group or panel discussions that include diverse representatives.

TOTAL QUALITY MANAGEMENT

Total quality management (TQM) is a quality management philosophy that promises to meet the needs of all customers within an organization. TQM promotes continuous improvement and quality in all aspects of an organization. TQM's goals are to increase customer satisfaction, productivity, and profits through efficiency and cost reductions. TQM requires:

- Information regarding customers' needs and opinions.
- Involvement of staff at all levels in decision-making, goal setting, and problem solving.
- Management's commitment to empowering staff.
- Management's accountability through active leadership and participation.
- Teamwork with incentives and rewards for accomplishments.

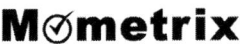

The focus of TQM is on working together to identify and solve problems, rather than assigning blame, through an organizational culture that focuses on the needs of the customers.

THE COST OF QUALITY

While TQM focuses on meeting needs of all customers within an organization, it is also equally important to consider the cost of quality. The cost of quality is a concept introduced by Philip Crosby with two components: the cost of good quality and the cost of poor quality. Crosby suggests that conformance to standards is equivalent to high quality and is less wasteful than the rework involved with poor quality or non-conformance to standards.

14 POINTS FOR QUALITY MANAGEMENT

W. Edwards Deming developed 14 Points for Quality Management to assist Japan with its industrial revival after World War II, and they are now widely applied to managing quality in healthcare organizations. The points are:

- **Create constancy**: Keep focus on the purpose — improvement of products and/or services.
- **Develop a new philosophy**: Provide effective training to ensure that things are done right the first time without delays, errors, or inefficiencies.
- **Stop depending on mass inspections**: Eliminate the need for mass inspections by building quality into procedures, so that inspection is at the beginning of a process, instead of at the end, in order to prevent problems.
- **Stop focusing on profits**: Assure staff that quality is more important than price.
- **Improve constantly**: Always strive to improve every process and decrease costs through organization-wide efforts at all levels.
- **Institute training**: Provide regular training to all levels of employees to ensure people understand their responsibilities and how to improve.
- **Adopt effective leadership**: Increase productivity by assisting those who need help to achieve their work goals.
- **Eliminate fear**: Communicate effectively, so employees feel secure and not fearful of punitive action.
- **Reduce barriers**: Encourage interdisciplinary teamwork, rather than competition between areas or departments within an organization.
- **Eliminate slogans**: Provide staff with methods to improve, rather than exhortations about the need for improvement.
- **Eliminate numerical quotas/goals**: Focus on quality, rather than numbers, as a means to improve productivity.
- **Remove barriers to pride of workmanship**: Encourage the efforts of staff. Eliminate annual rating or merit systems.
- **Provide and encourage education**: Provide ongoing educational programs for all levels of employees within an organization to foster a desire for self-improvement.
- **Outline management's commitment to transforming the workplace**: Actively encourage staff to constantly strive to follow the 14 Points and do the best that they can.

Continuous Quality Improvement (CQI)

Continuous Quality Improvement (CQI) is a type of multidisciplinary management philosophy that applies to all aspects of an organization, including medicine, purchasing, and human resources. Epidemiologic research skills are applied to analyze multiple types of events (data collection, analysis, outcomes, and action plans) because they are based on solid scientific methods. Multi-disciplinary planning brings valuable insights from various perspectives, because strategies used in one context can often be applied to another. All departments are increasingly concerned with cost-effectiveness as the costs of medical care continue to rise, so the quality professional is not isolated, but is part of the whole, facing similar concerns as those in other disciplines. Disciplines are often interrelated in their functions. For example, the Human Resources Department hires personnel, but other staff monitor and train them for compliance with organizational standards.

Continuous Quality Improvement (CQI) emphasizes the organization, systems and processes within a medical institution, rather than individuals. CQI recognizes internal customers (staff) and external customers (patients) and uses data to improve processes. Foundational concepts of CQI include the following:

- Most processes can be improved
- Quality and success are meeting or exceeding internal and external customers' needs and expectations
- Problems relate to processes
- Variations in processes lead to variations in results
- Change can be in small steps

Tools for CQI include the following:

- Scientific method of experimentation and documentation
- Brainstorming
- Multi-voting
- Charts and diagrams
- Storyboarding
- Meetings

Developing an Intradisciplinary and Interdisciplinary Curriculum

The CPHQ should develop an intradisciplinary and interdisciplinary curriculum to improve patient outcomes and quality of care with the following steps:

- **Create**: Education can include formal classes, informal discussions as part of team meetings, handouts, and computer-assisted learning (especially for night shift workers). If time is lacking to personally develop different materials for each group on-site, ask the human resources department for help, or purchase customizable training materials.
- **Coordinate**: Consider the diverse needs of different groups and plan ways to provide education to all staff members on all shifts. Adjust work schedules, offer the same presentations at different times, and broadcast and record presentations for viewing by staff that cannot attend live presentations.
- **Implement**: Schedule training to ensure the staff has adequate notice, patient care is covered, and schedules are adjusted so all can participate.
- **Evaluate**: Ask each participant to complete a course evaluation form. Evaluate the ongoing education process and make periodic evaluations of outcomes to ensure goals were met.

PROCESS IMPROVEMENT

Quality process improvement's primary principle is that advances can be accomplished in small, incremental steps. In large organizations with many employees, process improvement is a formal process. In small organizations or individual departments, the basic procedures are the same, but modify procedures accordingly for fewer employees. Begin continuous quality process improvement by identifying one process that needs improvement. For example:

1. Clearly state the problem: "Poor telephone service leads to dropped calls and miscommunications between the lab pathologist and the operating room surgeon regarding cancer biopsy patients."
2. Contact various telephone service providers and compare features.
3. Choose the better telephone service.

When the steps to improving the telephone process are completed, immediately pick another project for improvement. Multiple continuous improvement projects are in process at the same time.

CONDUCTING AN EDUCATIONAL NEEDS ASSESSMENT

Follow these steps for an educational needs assessment:

- Review job descriptions to determine all staff's educational qualifications and certifications to determine what, realistically, they should be expected to know about the subject (e.g., infection control).
- Review existing job orientation and training materials to determine what staff members have already been taught about performance improvement.
- Conduct meetings with staff in different departments to brainstorm areas of concern and potential training needs.
- Meet with team leaders and department heads for their input about the need for infection control education.
- Pretest staff with short quizzes that ask about standard performance improvement methods to determine their basic knowledge.
- Provide questionnaires to staff to obtain information about their own perceptions of what they know or need to know about performance improvement.
- Make direct observations of staff as they work.

DEVELOPING GOALS, MEASURABLE OBJECTIVES, AND LESSON PLANS FOR EDUCATION

The performance improvement team chooses an education topic, then the CPHQ develops goals, measurable objectives with strategies, and lesson plans. Focus the class on one area, e.g., proper hand washing technique. Do not make a survey course covering a broad area, like infection control in general. For example:

- **Goal**: To increase compliance with hand hygiene standards in the ICU.
- **Objectives**:
    - Capture potential students' attention through posters
    - Maintain 100% compliance with hand hygiene standards at 2 weeks, 1-month, and 2-month intervals after training
- **Strategy**:
    - Hang posters in all nursing units, staff rooms, and utility rooms by March 1
    - Develop digital slide presentation and obtain intranet access for class by May 24

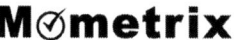

- o Conduct four classes at different times from May 25–31
- o Distribute hand washing kits
- **30-minute lesson plan**:
  - o Discussion: Why do we need 100% compliance? (5 min)
  - o Slide Presentation: The Case for Hand Hygiene (10 min)
  - o Discussion: What did you learn? (5 min)
  - o Demonstrate correct hand washing technique (5 min)
  - o Culture samples to show bacterial reduction (5 min)

APPLYING PRINCIPLES OF ADULT LEARNING TO EDUCATIONAL STRATEGIES

Adults come to work with a wealth of life and employment experiences. Their attitudes toward education vary considerably, but there are basic principles of adult learning and typical characteristics of adult learners that every instructor must consider when strategizing. Adult learners tend to be:

- **Practical and goal-oriented**:
  - o Provide overviews or summaries and examples.
  - o Use collaborative discussions with problem-solving exercises.
- **Self-directed**:
  - o Provide active involvement and ask for input.
  - o Allow different options for achieving the goal.
- **Knowledgeable**:
  - o Respect their life experiences and prior education.
  - o Validate their knowledge and ask for feedback.
  - o Relate new material to information with which they are already familiar.
- **Relevancy-oriented**:
  - o Explain how new information will apply on the job.
  - o Clearly identify objectives.
- **Motivated**:
  - o Provide certificates of professional advancement and/or continuing education credit when possible.

DETERMINING APPROPRIATE TEACHING APPROACHES

Consider audience size when planning presentations for the following reasons:

- Student participation is more difficult in a large class because there is no time for all to speak individually. Break the class into small discussion groups or pairs for part of the class time to increase participation. Focus the discussions so that students stay on task.
- For small groups, place chairs in a circle or sit around a table to allow students to look at each other and have more active discussions than if they sit in rows.
- Online virtual classes vary considerably in size, depending on the type of presentation and whether or not scores and replies are automated or posted by the instructor. If the online group is large, set up a chat room to facilitate the exchange of ideas.

UTILIZATION OF HANDOUTS

Handouts are fixtures in classes, but many end up in the wastebasket without ever being read. Follow these tips to provide useful handouts that will be read:

- Avoid slide show notes that repeat everything in the presentation; just summarize the main points.
- Distributing handouts immediately prior to a discussion ensures that most of the class will be looking at the handout instead of the speaker. Place handouts in a folder or binder. Distribute them before class so people can peruse them in advance, or as students leave the class.
- Use handouts to provide guidance or worksheets for small group discussions.
- Try poster handouts (with drawings or pictures) that can be placed on bulletin boards on the nursing units.
- Use an easily readable font, like Times New Roman 12-point, and avoid the use of smudged copies of newspaper articles or small print text.

CONSIDERATIONS REGARDING THE PHYSICAL LEARNING ENVIRONMENT

When considering the appropriate audiovisuals and handout materials for a course, keep the physical environment in mind for the following factors:

- Everyone in the room must be able to hear and see. For a small room, a television screen will suffice, but use a projection screen for an auditorium.
- Turn off the overhead lights and cover windows for low-resolution projectors. Flicking lights on and off during a presentation is very distracting. Use a small portable light at the podium, or use an alternate presentation format.
- Slide presentation or other presentations that include text must be of sufficient font size to be read from the back of the room.

ENSURING APPROPRIATE AND CURRENT CONTENT IN EDUCATIONAL MATERIALS

The CPHQ cannot produce all educational materials personally, so give careful consideration to the following factors:

- **Price** for educational materials ranges from free government issue to thousands of dollars for proprietary software. Decide if audiovisuals are needed, an entire course, or a series of courses. Consider the budget and then look for material within those monetary constraints online. The CDC, the Department of Labor, libraries, and universities often have text, posters, handouts, slide presentations, and videos available for free download.
- **Quality** varies considerably, so consider the goals and objectives before choosing materials. Trust sites with .gov and .org in their addresses more than blogs or sites with advertising. Only distribute the materials if they cover all needed information in a clear and engaging manner. Find at least two reputable sources that agree on the same information.
- **Currency** is an accreditation requirement. If the material will soon be outdated because of regulatory changes, ensure it can be replaced, and tell staff when to expect updates. Cite research published within the last five years.

Approaches to Teaching

There are many approaches to teaching, so the CPHQ must recognize the most appropriate format and plan for flexible class times, so patient care is not diminished:

- **Educational workshops** are conducted with small groups, allowing for maximum participation, and are especially good for demonstrations and practice sessions.
- **Lectures** are for academic or detailed information, but question and answer sessions and discussion are limited. An effective lecture includes audiovisual support.
- **Discussions** are best with small groups so the audience can actively participate in problem solving.
- **One-on-one instruction** is especially helpful for targeted or remedial instruction in procedures for individuals.
- **Computer/Internet modules** are good for independent learners and night shift staff.

Measuring Performance Improvement Training Effectiveness with Learner Outcomes

When the CPHQ plans an educational offering (class, online module, workshop, manuals, brochures), he or she identifies the desired **learner outcomes** from the very beginning, so that the learners are aware of the expectations. The subject matter of the educational material and the learner outcomes are directly related. For example, if the CPHQ teaches a class on environmental decontamination, then one learner outcome is: "By the end of this class, the learner will know the difference between disinfectants and antiseptics." There may be one or multiple learner outcomes. At the end of the learning experience, determine if the learner outcomes have been achieved by a survey. Ask learners if they felt they achieved the learner outcomes. Learners give valuable feedback and guidance to the CPHQ, even if they are not as familiar with the material as the CPHQ.

Behavior Modification and Compliance Rate

Educational efforts must be **evaluated**, like all interventions, for effectiveness. Two determinants of effectiveness are measures of behavior modification and compliance rates.

- **Behavior modification** involves thorough observation and measurement, identifying behavior that needs to be changed and then planning and instituting interventions to modify that behavior. Procedures a quality professional can use include demonstrations of appropriate behavior, reinforcement, and monitoring until new behavior is adopted consistently. This is especially important to change longstanding procedures and habits of behavior.
- **Compliance rates** are determined by observation at intervals and on multiple occasions. Outcomes are another measure of compliance; that is, if education is intended to improve patient safety and decrease infection rates and that occurs, it is a good indication that there is compliance. Calculate compliance rates by determining the number of events/procedures and degree of compliance through observation or record review.

Key Concepts of Quality Care

The key concepts of quality care should be communicated to all members of the organization through in-service training, workshops, newsletters, fact sheets, and team meetings. Quality care is:

- **Appropriate** to needs and follows best practice standards
- **Accessible** to everyone, despite financial, cultural, or other barriers
- **Competent**, with well-trained practitioners who adhere to standards
- **Coordinated** among all healthcare providers
- **Effective** in achieving outcomes, based on the current state of medical knowledge
- **Efficient** in its methods for achieving the desired outcomes
- **Preventive**, allowing for early detection and prevention of problems
- **Respectful**, so that the individual patient's needs are given primary importance
- **Safe**, so that the organization is free of hazards or dangers that put patients, visitors, and staff at risk
- **Timely**, ensuring the correct care is provided on time
- **Equitable**, ensuring that the type of care provided is consistent amongst all
- **Patient-centered**, ensuring that both the patient experience and outcomes are positive

Encouraging Use of Internal Resources and the Expertise of Others

Assisting staff to understand and use internal resources and the expertise of others requires a commitment of time and effort:

- Coach others on methods of **collaboration**. Provide handouts about effective communication strategies. Model collaboration with the staff being coached.
- Conduct **team meetings** for departments, where collaboration is modeled, and suggest the need for outside expertise to help with patient care planning. Initiate discussions about resources that are available within the facility (e.g., medical library, university affiliates, in-house trainers, bilingual staff, and expert users) and the community (e.g., public health, emergency medical services, Red Cross, immigrant settlement services, women's groups, and disease-specific support groups).
- Select diverse teams that reflect the population served within a geographical area, also known as the catchment area, or invite **subject matter experts** (SMEs) to mentor teams when needed.

Departmental Budgets

Types of Budgets

A departmental budget is part of a larger organizational budget. The CPHQ must understand the different types of budgets used in healthcare, in order to participate in financial management:

- **Operating budget**: The operating budget consists of revenue and costs (both fixed and variable). It is used for daily operations, and includes general expenses, such as salaries, education, insurance, maintenance, depreciation, debts, and profit.
- **Capital budget**: The capital budget determines which capital projects (such as remodeling, repairing, and purchasing of equipment or buildings) will be allocated funding for the year. These capital expenditures are usually based on cost-benefit analysis and prioritization of needs.

- **Cash balance budget**: The cash balance budget projects cash balances for a specific future time period, including all operating and capital budget items.
- **Master budget**: The master budget combines operating, capital, and cash balance budgets, and any specialized or area-specific budgets.

Different Approaches to Departmental Budgets

Most departmental budgets are operational, but a number of different approaches can be used:

- **Fixed/forecast**: Revenue and expenses are forecasted for the entire budget period and budget items are fixed.
- **Flexible**: Estimates are made regarding anticipated changes in revenue and expenses, and both fixed and variable costs are identified.
- **Zero-based**: All cost centers are re-evaluated each budget period to determine if they should be funded or eliminated, partially or completely.
- **Responsibility center**: Budgeting is by cost center, with one person holding overall responsibility.
- **Program**: Organizational programs are identified, and revenues and costs for each program are budgeted.
- **Appropriations**: Government funds are requested and disbursed through appropriations.
- **Continuous/rolling**: Periodic updates to the budget, including revenues, costs, and volume, are done prior to the next budget cycle.

Developing and Managing Departmental Budgets

Once the departmental budget is developed and established, budget management must occur on an ongoing basis to ensure that financial targets are met in relation to strategic goals. Management includes:

- **Accountability**: The budget team should include managers and directors who expect excellence.
- **Controlling expenses**: This is especially important for departments that do not produce income directly.
- **Monitoring costs in relation to best practice benchmarks**: One goal of budget management is to strive to match benchmarks.
- **Developing corrective action plans**: Any variances in the budget should be accounted for within a week and corrective actions taken.
- **Using a balanced scorecard**: Various measurements, both quantitative and qualitative, are used to manage cost containment strategies.
- **Recognizing quality**: Rewards for achieving benchmarks should be built into the budgeting process. In some cases, this may be a bonus payout.

Financial Management

Financial management is a part of strategic planning, in which the department demonstrates how its resources will be allocated, usually for a one-year period. Financial management includes:

- Developing and assigning budget items
- Monitoring expenditures
- Analysis
- Reporting

Sound financial management is based on the best utilization of costs in relation to revenues and outcomes. Objectives of financial management include:

- Developing a quantitative record of plans
- Allowing for evaluation of financial performance
- Controlling costs
- Providing information to increase cost awareness

The budget must be linked to daily operations and integrated with strategic vision, mission, goals, and objectives. Those with vested interests in the budget should participate in its planning. Monitoring should be ongoing to allow for feedback and modifications as necessary.

Activity-Based Costing (ABC) System

The activity-based costing (ABC) system is an accounting system that focuses on the costs of resources necessary for a process or service. There are some differences between ABC and traditional accounting, which is a cash-based system where the bookkeeper enters revenues when they are received and expenses when they are paid, so that revenues and expenses are not necessarily related. By contrast, ABC is an accrual system, where the bookkeeper enters revenues when they are earned and expenses as they are incurred, so that revenues and expenses are more closely tied. The basic formula for ABC is to divide the total output into total cost to arrive at a unit cost. The general steps to ABC are:

- Identify activities involved in processes and outputs.
- Calculate cost of resources for activities, including direct costs, indirect costs, and administrative (general overhead) costs.
- Identify all outputs related to activities and utilization of resources.
- Allocate costs of activities to outputs; cost drivers are costs of resources related to activities.

Financial Costs Related to Quality Management

Performance improvement is not without costs, and these must be considered carefully when doing a cost analysis. Financial costs related to quality management include the following:

- **Error-free costs**, which are the costs of all processes, services, equipment, time, materials, and staffing necessary to provide a product or process that is without error from its outset. A process that is error-free is relatively stable in terms of pre-established guidelines.
- **Cost of quality** (COQ) includes costs associated with identifying and correcting errors, defects or failures in processes and planning, and costs of poor quality (COPQ).
- **Conformance costs** are those costs related to preventing errors, such as monitoring and evaluation. This may include education, maintenance, pilot testing, and analysis.
- **Nonconformance costs** are those related to errors, failures, and defects. These include adverse events (such as infections), poor patient access due to staff shortages, appointment and surgery cancellations, lost time, duplications of service, and malpractice fines.

Justifying Expenditures
Cost-Benefit Analysis

A cost-benefit analysis uses the average cost of an event and the cost of an intervention to demonstrate savings. For example: According to the CDC, a surgical site infection caused by *Staphylococcus aureus* results in an average of 12 additional days of hospitalization and costs $27,000. (In actuality, the cost varies widely from one institution to another, so use local data if it benefits the institution's case.) If an institution averages 10 surgical site infections annually, the cost is 10 x $27,000 = **$270,000** annually. If the proposed interventions include:

- New software for surveillance ($10,000)
- An additional staff person ($65,000 salary + $15,000 benefits)
- Increased staff education, including materials ($2000)
- Then the total intervention cost would be $10,000 + $65,000 + $15,000 + $2000 = **$92,000.00**

If the goal were to decrease infections by 50%, to 5 infections per year, the savings would be 5 × $27,000 = **$135,000.** Subtract the intervention cost from the savings to obtain the annual cost benefit: $135,000 – $92,000 = **$43,000**

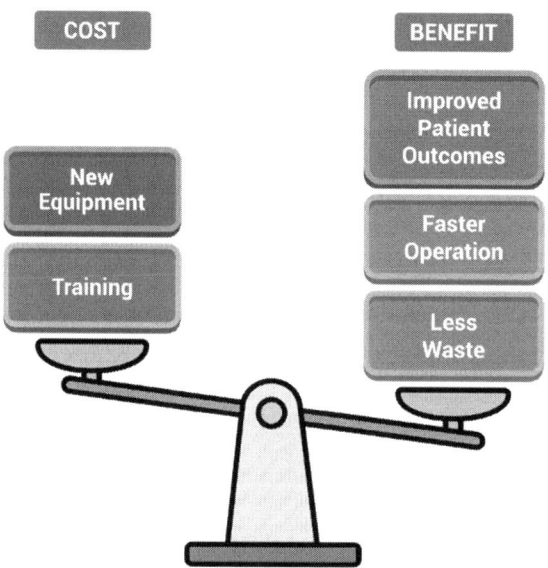

Cost-Effective Analysis, Efficacy Studies, and Incremental Cost-Effectiveness Ratio

A cost-effective analysis measures the effectiveness of an intervention rather than its monetary savings.

For example: Each year, 2 million nosocomial infections result in 90,000 deaths and $6.7 billion in additional health costs. From that perspective, decreasing infections should reduce costs, but there are human savings in suffering as well, and it is difficult to place a dollar value on that. If each infection adds about 12 days to hospitalization, then a reduction in infections by 5 would be calculated as 5 × 12 = 60 fewer patient infection days.

Efficacy studies compare a series of cost-benefit analyses to determine the intervention with the best cost-benefit. Efficacy studies can also be used for process or product evaluation.

For example: A study is conducted to determine the infection rates of four different types of catheters. The catheter type that results in the fewest infections saves the most money and infection days.

Incremental cost-effectiveness ratio is the difference between a cost change and an outcome change.

Cost-Utility Analysis

Cost-utility analysis (CUA) is essentially a sub-type of cost-effective analysis, but CUA is more complex and its results are more difficult to quantify and use to justify expense. Cost-utility analysis measures the benefit of an intervention to society in general, such as decreasing teenage pregnancies. Often, the standards used to quantify CUA are somewhat subjective. CUA compares a variety of outcomes (e.g., increased life expectancy and decreased suffering) in relation to the quality-adjusted-life year (QALY). A health condition is assigned a number on a scale—referred to as its utility—in which 1 represents normal health and 0 represents death. When calculating outcomes with CUA, an intervention is evaluated on whether or not it increases the utility score, and thereby increases life expectancy or improves life circumstances by X number of years. Thus, the CUA results are not expressed as monetary values, but rather as societal values.

Cost Allocation

One type of cost analysis involves cost allocation. With almost all expenditures, there are direct costs and indirect costs. For example, the salary of a team leader is a direct cost. Indirect costs are those related to accounting and human resources. To determine cost allocation, the CPHQ must use line-item budget format. List each item with its unit cost or cost per unit of service. Determine direct costs and indirect costs. Generally, direct costs benefit just one department or service, while indirect costs are shared costs, such as the cost of custodial services. Thus, a percentage of the indirect cost is allocated to a department based on its utilization.

For example: If team leaders represent 5% of the total employees, then 5% of indirect employee costs would be allocated to this line item. Remember, there are many departments and services involved in indirect costs. To arrive at a true unit cost, account for all of these costs.

Developing Performance Improvement Plans

To develop a performance improvement plan, follow these steps:

1. Design the process	Choose an approach that focuses on quality planning, control, and improvement. Assemble a team. Establish a process based on data. Identify customers. Assess the organization's ability to implement a plan. Include training needs and resources in the initial design.
2. Design the plan	Plan strategically for organization-wide participation and collaborative activities, which may be department or discipline-specific, or interdisciplinary. Make the plan consistent with the organization's vision and mission statements, and its goals and objectives. Include performance expectations and measurements.
3. Plan for implementation	Write the plan, including a definition of quality; standards of care; guidelines for patient safety; benchmarks; and outcome measurements. Educate leadership and staff.

The CPHQ must resolve these issues to develop a performance improvement plan:

- **Leadership roles**: Delineate the roles of the key leaders in writing, beginning at the highest level (such as the Chief Executive Officer), so that their responsibilities are clear.
- **Terminology related to quality**: Use consistent terminology in all documents and activities. Decide whether to refer to quality management (QM), quality resource management (QRM), continuous quality improvement (CQI) or some other acronym.

- **Accountability structure**: Determine who will sit on the quality council. Its members set priorities regarding staff time, finances, and resources, and ensure accountability. The quality council should be one structure, which may require the integration of existing bodies or the creation of a new entity. The quality council oversees the plan, reports to the governing board, and communicates with leaders at all levels.

DOCUMENTATION AND PAPERWORK

As part of the process of developing a performance improvement plan, the CPHQ should prioritize the following documentation and paperwork:

- **Create a flow chart**: Include the complete organizational structure, with all the participating councils, teams, and lines of authority and communication. Provide a copy for all team members.
- **Integrate policies, statements, and plans**: Update documentation across the organization, so that all use the same terminology (e.g., customers or consumers, public or non-staff). Make a consistent glossary of definitions.
- **Link goals with performance improvement activities**: All performance activities must reference the organization's specific strategic goals or objectives and its mission and vision statements. If there is a disparity, then either the vision and mission statements must be adjusted, or the focus of the improvement activities must be changed. The mission and vision statements are central to quality healthcare planning. Plan all activities with the intention of meeting established goals and objectives.

WRITING PERFORMANCE IMPROVEMENT PLANS

Document every performance improvement plan in writing. Tailor the written plan to its purpose. It may be brief if it is intended primarily as a teaching tool to guide staff, but if it is intended as a tool for implementation, it must be a comprehensive document that outlines in detail all of the different aspects of the performance improvement plan. A detailed plan must include:

- A statement of commitment
- A clear outline of authority and responsibility
- An explanation of the infrastructure
- An outline of the flow of information

The organization may require a written plan for its state licensure or participation in federal plans. Obtain a copy of the specific state and federal requirements, and ensure the plan corresponds to them exactly. The goals and objectives of a quality plan must clearly relate to the organization's overall strategic goals and objectives. Outline the structure and design of leadership and teams and delineate their responsibilities. Get approvals from all interested parties and keep the originals on file with the document.

Team Reporting and Structures

A performance improvement plan requires the CPHQ to do the following as they relate to team reporting and structures:

- **Establish a reporting structure and calendar**: Performance improvement activities are usually reported on a monthly basis or another regular, frequent schedule. Distribute a detailed written report and present a synopsis at team and management meetings. Remind the directors and managers to disseminate the monthly report through staff meetings. Post a calendar, which clearly indicates a proposed timeline for improvements, and lists regular meeting times.
- **Determine the team structures**: A number of different teams may be necessary, depending on the model selected. Assign the teams very specific functions, such as patient assessment, clinical improvement, and operations improvement. Determine which teams should be interdisciplinary, which teams should be department-specific, and who should be included.

Addressing Educational Needs and Team Training

A performance improvement plan must also address educational needs and team training recommendations:

- **Identify the specific educational needs of leaders and staff**: Decide who requires education. State the educational needs of each group of participants, and what the organization can appropriately provide. List the means for providing this education. For example, an organization can provide on-site computer training during regular work hours, but staff must renew their CPR and First Aid certification off-site, in their own time, through an independent third-party provider, such as the Red Cross. Create an executive summary and detailed plan for all those in leadership positions, beginning with the governing board, so they thoroughly understand the performance improvement plan, its data collection, measurement, and analysis.
- **Plan for training teams**: Relate general training to team structure, team functions, and team leadership. Ensure the individual team members get training for their specific roles, so teams work consistently.

Functions and Models

Functions are the specialized activities of a system. Functions include not only patient care, but also governance, management, and support. If function is the focus, rather than individual departments, it integrates services and makes patient care the priority, rather than the departmental processes themselves. Identify functions by analyzing patient tracers, performance measures, cost data, reviews, and claims data.

Model (or methodology): This refers to the guide for a performance improvement plan, such as FOCUS, PDCA, 10-Step Benchmarking, QIP, or Six Sigma. Review all models and pick the one that best meets the needs of the organization and will be accepted by all interested parties. Part of one's decision relates to available resources and the degree of commitment the organization has to performance improvement.

Communication

ACTIVE LISTENING

Therapeutic communication begins with respect for the patient and his or her family. Make a personal introduction, use the patient's name, and listen intently. **Active listening** is critical in creating a therapeutic environment that fosters teamwork and change:

- **Use open-ended questions**: "Is there anything you'd like to discuss?"
- **Acknowledge comments** by nodding or stating, "Yes, I understand."
- **Reflect** statements back (use sparingly):
  - Patient: "I hate it here!"
  - Staff: "You hate it here?"
- Make **observations**:
  - "You are shaking."
  - "You seem worried."
- **Recognize** the patient's feelings:
  - Patient: "I want to go home."
  - Staff: "It must be hard to be away from your family and friends."
- **Allow silence** and observe nonverbal behavior, rather than force conversation.
- **Provide information** as honestly and completely as possible about the patient's condition, treatment, and procedures.

PROMOTING CARING AND SUPPORTIVE ENVIRONMENTS

Therapeutic communication phrases that support patient care include the following:

- Express **implied messages**:
  - Patient: "This treatment is too much trouble."
  - Staff: "You think the treatment isn't helping you?"
- **Explore a topic**, but allow the patient to terminate the discussion without further probing:
  - "I'd like to hear how you feel about that."
- Indicate **reality**:
  - Patient: "Someone is screaming."
  - Staff: "That sound was an ambulance siren."
- **Comment on distortions** without directly agreeing or disagreeing:
  - Patient: "That nurse promised I wouldn't have any shot!"
  - Staff: "Really? That's surprising because this medicine can only be given as an injection."
- **Work together**:
  - "Maybe if we talk about this, we can figure out a way to make the treatment easier for you."
- **Seek validation**:
  - "Do you feel better now?"
  - "Did the medication help you breathe better?"

AVOIDING NON-THERAPEUTIC COMMUNICATION

While using therapeutic communication is important, it is equally important to **avoid interjecting non-therapeutic communication**, which blocks effective communication. Avoid the following:

- Meaningless **clichés**:
    - "Don't worry. Everything will be fine."
    - "Isn't it a nice day?"

- Providing **unsought advice**:
    - "You should…" or "The best thing to do is…" Patients are more likely to accept if they ask for it.
    - Provide facts and encourage the patient to reach a decision.

- **Inappropriate approval** that prevents the patient from expressing true feelings or concerns:
    - Patient: "I shouldn't cry when Mommy goes home."
    - Staff: "That's right! You're a big boy!"

- **Asking for explanations** of behaviors that are not directly related to patient care and that require analysis and explanation of feelings:
    - "Why are you crying?"

- **Agreeing with, rather than accepting and responding to**, the patient's statements, making it more difficult for the patient to change his or her statement or opinion later:
    - "I agree with you," or "You're right."

Additional examples of non-therapeutic communication include the following:

- **Negative judgments**: "You should stop arguing with the nurses."
- **Devaluing the patient's feelings**: "Everyone gets upset at times."
- **Disagreeing directly**: "That can't be true," or "I think you are wrong."
- **Defending against criticism**: "The doctor is not being rude, he's just very busy today."
- **Changing the subject** to avoid dealing with uncomfortable topics:
    - Patient: "I'm never going to get well."
    - Staff: "Your parents will be here in just a few minutes."
- **Inappropriate literal responses**, even as a joke, especially if the patient is at all confused or having difficulty expressing ideas:
    - Patient: "There are bugs crawling under my skin."
    - Staff: "I'll get some bug spray."
- **Challenging to establish reality**, which often just increases confusion and frustration: "If you were dying, you wouldn't be able to yell and kick!"

INTERNAL COMMUNICATION DUTIES

The quality professional fulfills organization-wide communication duties by:

- **Reviewing communications** related to process improvement, reports, and feedback to determine if:
    o The governing body and staff are familiar with strategic goals and successful improvement processes.
    o Each staff member is aware of his or her personal responsibilities for patient safety.
- **Providing communications** organization-wide, in an easily accessible format, such as:
    o Ensuring policies and procedures manuals are online.
    o Making calendars with timelines for reports and other process improvement activities.
    o Sending email reminders.
    o Giving regular reports and updates at department, management, and team meetings.
    o Communications are in a variety of formats, such as newsletters, emails, screensavers, and FAQ sheets.

Teams

PERFORMANCE IMPROVEMENT TEAM

A **performance improvement team** is a group of people working together to achieve a goal, like writing a clinical action plan to make workflows more efficient. Performance improvement activities almost always involve a team or teams of staff because of the complexity of healthcare organizations. Rarely is one department solely responsible for outcomes, except in very specialized work. Tracer methodology is a method that looks at the continuum of care a patient receives from admission to post-discharge. When determining the composition of the performance improvement team, use tracer methodology to ensure there is at least one representative from all groups that participate in patient care on the team. Teamwork requires a considerable time and training commitment. Performance improvement initiatives require teams to:

- Improve outcomes through a common purpose
- Utilize staff expertise
- Contribute various perspectives
- Facilitate a participative management style
- Improve acceptance of processes that impact work practice
- Manage complexity, where many participants are involved
- Increase organization-wide acceptance of change
- Combat resistance to change

ADVANTAGES

Advantages of developing performance improvement teams include the following:

- **Individual**: Team members have the opportunity to develop new skills, share their expertise, utilize their creativity, increase their personal autonomy, influence decisions, and improve their job satisfaction. Working in teams often increases the team members' respect for other disciplines and members.
- **Administrative**: The organization's administration benefits when it has increased flexibility to facilitate, rather than direct. Delegating performance improvement to teams means administrators have fewer time constraints, increased staff support, better utilization of skills, and improved productivity. Utilizing teams frees administrators from many time-consuming tasks, allowing for better overall management.
- **Organization-wide**: The organization benefits by more continuity, customer satisfaction, cost efficiency, improved productivity, more efficient accountability, decreased staff turnover, and an improved ability to deal with staff turnover. Teams benefit the entire organization because they are more suited to dealing with complexity than individuals.

TEAM STRUCTURE

The appropriate team structure is very important in performance improvement because creating a team does not, in itself, assure teamwork. The team must be comprised of individuals whose skills complement each other and who have a shared purpose, because outcomes depend on the collaborative efforts of the group, rather than individuals within the group. Accordingly, the collective team is accountable for outcomes, rather than individuals. When creating teams, consider these important elements:

- **Size**: Teams with less than 10 members are most effective.
- **Skills**: Team members should have complementary skills that encompass the technical, problem solving, decision-making, and interpersonal aspects of the problem.

- **Performance goals**: Allow teams a degree of autonomy to produce action plans for performance improvement, based on strategic goals and objectives.
- **Unified approach**: Create the teams according to the model of performance improvement chosen but allow them some flexibility in working together.
- **Accountability**: Make the team members collectively accountable, rather than individually accountable.

Teams may come together permanently, temporarily, virtually, or naturally (through closely related work functions). Regardless of the format, teams should be evaluated by considering the productivity, satisfaction, and individual growth of team members.

CROSS-FUNCTIONAL TEAMS

Cross-functional teams are sometimes called interdisciplinary. Cross-functional teams are comprised of individuals with various skill levels or from different disciplines, who work together to accomplish one or more functions. An ad hoc team operates for a short time to accomplish specific goals. A permanent team is a regular part of continuous performance improvement. Cross-functional teams are particularly useful when it is required to:

- Develop new processes.
- Implement organization-wide performance changes or technology.
- Control costs and increase the cost-benefit ratio.
- Deal with problems or performance activities that cross disciplines.
- Access a broad range of expertise and skills.

To ensure the success of performance improvement activities:

- Select team members with the correct mix of abilities.
- Clearly outline the roles for the team members.
- List the expected outcomes.
- Provide adequate training to assist cross-functional team members in working together as a unit.

SELF-DIRECTED WORK TEAMS

Self-directed work teams are groups of individuals working together to achieve a common goal, such as improving a process or producing a product. While the members may be trained cross-functionally, they usually have individual functions within the group. Usually, the teams have an assigned task or tasks for which they are accountable, but have the authority to manage the functions on their own, and make decisions without the direction of the administration. As with other types of teams, self-directed work teams may be ad hoc or permanent. Their degree of autonomy varies from one organization to another. Self-directed work teams may do the following:

- Plan and establish priorities
- Organize and manage budgets
- Manage work schedules and assignments
- Engage in problem-solving activities and make corrections
- Monitor and evaluate performance
- Coordinate with other teams or individuals
- Choose or hire team members

PERFORMANCE OVERSIGHT GROUP

The performance oversight group is often referred to as the quality council, steering council, or quality management committee. The governing board establishes the performance oversight group to coordinate all performance improvement activities. The group is usually drawn from administrative leaders, medical staff, and key personnel in various departments. The chairperson of the group is usually appointed by the President or Chief Executive Officer of the organization, and is approved by the medical staff and governing board. Part of the role of the facilitator is to:

- Inform the governing board of the need for the group
- Estimate/Calculate the cost of the group's activities
- Develop a preliminary list of group responsibilities
- Match responsibilities with the skills, knowledge, roles, and vision of group members
- Schedule regular meetings for the group, ranging from twice monthly to 10 times yearly
- Report the group's activities regularly to the governing board
- Document the group's performance improvement activities
- Maintain confidentiality of patient and practitioner information, in accordance with HIPAA

RESPONSIBILITIES

The performance oversight group has tremendous influence over the success of a performance improvement plan, so potential group members must be aware of their responsibilities and willing to participate. Disseminate preliminary information about performance improvement at meetings held to discuss the issues. The **responsibilities of the performance oversight group** are to:

- Develop, modify, and approve the performance improvement plan
- Establish priorities for initiatives, based on patient impact, data, and organizational objectives
- Select the types of teams needed, establish teams, and supervise them
- Plan methodologies to support action plans
- Review aggregate data, measurements of performance, and periodic summaries from teams
- Establish a confidential peer review policy
- Establish educational and training programs as needed
- Supervise a budget and make budgetary recommendations
- Evaluate the effectiveness of performance activities
- Provide summaries of achievement activities and progress toward goals

ROLES WITHIN A PERFORMANCE IMPROVEMENT TEAM

There are a number of key roles within a performance improvement team, and selecting the best-suited candidate to fill each role greatly influences the effectiveness of the team. The key roles are:

- **Facilitator** (Master Black Belt in Six Sigma): The facilitator is not a member of the team, but rather consults with or coaches the team members, helps to build team skills, and keeps the team focused. The facilitator may:
    - Provide training
    - Assist the team leader or team members
    - Receive input from team members
    - Evaluate consensus
    - Provide feedback
    - Summarize outcomes

- **Team leader** (Black Belt in Six Sigma): This team leader is a member of the team who provides direction, but is not individually responsible for decision-making, or the overall effectiveness of the team's efforts. Often, team leaders are middle managers that coach, rather than direct, members of the team. The team leader may:
    o Prepare and conduct meetings
    o Assign activities
    o Evaluate progress
    o Coordinate with other teams
    o Communicate with the facilitator
    o Document meetings and activities
- **Team member** (Green Belt in Six Sigma): The team member is a critical part of the team because this person performs many of the actual hands-on activities related to team responsibilities. The team member may:
    o Attend all meetings
    o Provide input for the agenda
    o Assist the team leader
    o Share expertise
    o Communicate with other team members
    o Complete specific assignments
    o Propose projects
    o Measure
    o Collect data
    o Recommend actions
- **Secretary/Recorder**: The Secretary is responsible for keeping minutes and creating other reports or documents as needed by the team. This position may become the responsibility of one person or may be done on a rotating basis by various team members. Careful documentation and reporting are a necessary function of teams, so that their progress can be evaluated and reports disseminated to management.
- **Timekeeper**: The timekeeper monitors the time spent in meetings and keeps people on track, so that meeting times are well spent, and do not exceed scheduled times. This position is often rotated among team members.
- **Sponsor**: The sponsor may be the quality council as a whole, or a key leader with an interest in the particular activities of a team. The sponsor is not involved in the day-to-day activity of the group, but receives regular reports regarding the team's activities. The sponsor reviews the team's efforts and may provide guidance or direction. The sponsor maintains overall responsibility and accountability for the team effort, and has a primary role in the selection of projects and other members of the team. The sponsor ensures that all interested parties are informed, monitors decisions and activities, and has the authority to implement changes.

CHAMPIONS VS. PROCESS OWNERS

Champions are those individuals with a particular passion for or interest in the activities of a performance improvement team and are often instrumental in the creation and formation of the teams themselves, choosing the basic function of the team and the team members. Because members of organizations very often resist change, the champion has a pivotal role in providing leadership.

- The **process champion** is often a member of upper management with significant influence, who has the authority to make decisions, and the ability to communicate with top management and the governing board. The champion is often an individual with expertise in the area of focus and provides input when needed to drive the initiative forward.
- Champions can exist at different levels, so there may be **clinical champions** or **patient safety champions**—individuals who have made an effort to be informed and to promote performance improvement.

Process owners, on the other hand, are usually the team leaders, who are actively involved in supervising and/or carrying out the functions and activities of the team. Process owners are often key managers with knowledge and commitment to improvement.

BUILDING TEAMS

Leading, facilitating, and participating in performance improvement teams requires a thorough understanding of team-building dynamics. Teams may progress through several stages of development, as described by Tuckman's framework outlining team evolution: forming, storming, norming and performing. Each stage can be identified and optimized by understanding the following team-building dynamics:

- **Initial interactions**: The time when members define their roles and develop relationships, which determines if they are comfortable in the group. These initial interactions are comparable to the first stage of Tuckman's framework called **forming.**
- **Power issues**: The members observe the leader and determine who controls the meeting and how control is exercised; they begin to form alliances. As tension amongst the group begins to arise, the leader of the team must adjust their leadership style to accommodate and manage conflict. The conflict and division amongst the group is comparable to the second stage of Tuckman's framework called the **storming** phase.
- **Organizing**: Methods to achieve work are clarified and team members begin to work together, gaining respect for each other's contributions and working toward a common goal. It is at this time that the team is considered to be in the **norming** phase.
- **Team identification**: Interactions become less formal as members develop rapport, so members are more willing to help and support each other to achieve goals.
- **Excellence**: The team achieves success through a combination of good leadership, committed team members, clear goals, high standards, external recognition, a spirit of collaboration, and a shared commitment to the process. This is considered the **performing** stage.

It is equally important for healthcare quality professionals to understand the drivers of success and failure for a team. For a team to have long-term success, there are four factors to consider: cohesiveness, communication, clarity relating to roles, and clarity relating to goals. The absence of any one of these factors places the team's functionality and overall success at risk.

Leading Meetings

Good techniques for leading meetings include the following:

- **Scheduling**: Review the work schedules of those involved. Find the most convenient time for all attendees. Choose a place convenient and conducive to working together. Meeting rooms must have a round table to facilitate an equal exchange of ideas, or room to sit in a circle. Order computers, overhead projectors, whiteboards, a tape recorder, and any other necessary equipment.
- **Preparation**: Prepare a detailed agenda with a list of items for discussion and an approximate time limit for each. Email the minutes from the last meeting to attendees.
- **Conducting the meeting**: Introduce each item on the agenda and solicit input from all group members. Assign tasks to individual members based on their interest and part in the process. Summarize input and begin a tentative future agenda. Announce the time and place of the next meeting.
- **Observation**: Watch the interactions of team members, including verbal and nonverbal communication, and respond.

Preparing a Team Contract

Many problems that arise with teams are avoidable if the team members reach a consensus about their expectations before group work begins. Complete a team contract at the initial meeting. All members must participate. Team contracts include these sections:

- **Roles**: Delineate the specific responsibilities of each team member, including the leader.
- **Discussion**: Decide if meetings will be agenda-driven, follow Robert's rules, or open discussion.
- **Time**: State the amount of time that members are expected to commit to team activities, including attending meetings.
- **Conduct**: Clarify acceptable parameters for behavior, including those for the individuals and the group.
- **Conflict resolution**: Agree on triggers for conflict resolution and methods.
- **Reports**: List the types of reports, timeline, and responsibility for preparing the reports.
- **Consequences**: Clearly state the penalty for failure to follow the contract.

Delegating Tasks

Effective leaders delegate work. Leaders who take on too much of the workload cripple themselves. Failure to delegate shows an inherent distrust in team members. To delegate effectively, do the following:

- Assess the skills and available time of the team members; determine if a task is suitable for an individual.
- Assign tasks with clear instructions and a timeline; explain objectives and expectations.
- Ensure tasks are completed properly and on time by monitoring progress, but not by micromanaging.
- Review the final results and record outcomes.

Mentor, monitor, and provide feedback and intervention as necessary during this process, because the leader is ultimately responsible for the delegated work. While delegated tasks may not always be completed successfully, they represent learning opportunities for staff.

REFRAINING FROM DELEGATING TASKS

Delegation of tasks is central to working in teams, but the leader must decide which tasks to perform personally. Not every task can be delegated. Retain tasks related to strategic planning and management, such as the following:

- **Leadership**: Regardless of one's leadership style, ultimate authority and responsibility for teamwork is retained by the leader. Shared leadership duties lead to confusion and resentment on the part of team members.
- **Monitoring**: Control the process through effective monitoring to ensure all tasks are completed on time.
- **Discipline**: Deal with misconduct privately; do not discuss it with the group.
- **Strategic goals and planning**: The leader is responsible for keeping the goals in mind and working toward the organizational vision.
- **Communication**: Keep all members informed. Be available for consultation.
- **Outcomes assessment**: Direct the final performance review; debrief and disband personally.

MANAGEMENT'S LINES OF AUTHORITY AND ACCOUNTABILITY

The Joint Commission has established leadership standards that apply to healthcare organizations and help to establish management's lines of authority and accountability. Under these standards, leadership comprises the governing body, the Chief Executive Officer, senior managers, department leaders, leaders (both elected and appointed) of staff or departments, the Nursing Executive, and other nurse leaders. The governing body is ultimately responsible for all patient care rendered by all types of practitioners (physicians, nurses, laboratory staff, and support staff) within and under the jurisdiction of the organization. The governing body must clearly outline the lines of authority and accountability for others in management positions. Each level of management must establish performance standards and performance measurements, so that accountability becomes transparent, and is based on data that can be used to drive changes when needed, to bring about improved outcomes.

Evidence-Based Practice

EVIDENCE-BASED PRACTICE GUIDELINES (EBP)

Evidence-based practice guidelines (EBP) for such things as standing medication orders or antibiotic protocols are in common use, but decisions are often made based on studies that lack internal and/or external validity, or on expert opinion colored by personal bias, so the process of establishing evidence-based practice guidelines should be done systematically. One must base decisions on solid evidence as much as possible. Include those who resist the process in order to facilitate the acceptance of guidelines. Simply dispensing evidence-based practice guidelines often does not change practice. Consider how the change will be implemented. Decide if the guidelines are mandatory for standing orders, and to what degree individual practitioners can choose other options. Guidelines that are too rigid are counterproductive. In some cases, establishing guidelines may affect cost-reimbursement from third-party payers.

To implement evidence-based practice guidelines (EBP), focus on the following:

- **Topic/Methodology**: List possible interventions or treatments for review. Choose patient populations and settings. Determine significant outcomes. Outline search boundaries (journal titles and types of studies). Use studies published within the last five years, unless historical trends are needed.
- **Evidence review**: Review the literature. Critically analyze studies. Summarize the results, including pooled meta-analysis.
- **Expert judgment**: If the evidence review produces inadequate evidence, use recommendations from subject matter experts (SMEs). Acknowledge the SMEs' subjective evidence in the policy.
- **Policy considerations**: Weigh cost-effectiveness, access to care, insurance coverage, availability of qualified staff, and legal implications.
- **Policy**: Write a policy for the organization's P&P manual. Rank recommendations by letter, so that *A* is the highest rating, based on the quality of supporting evidence.
- **Review**: Submit completed policy for peer review before instituting it. Keep the authorizing signatures on file. Update and renew the policy at least every two years.

Leading and Facilitating Change

MOTIVATING STAFF

An organization's leaders must understand **staff's motivation** to increase productivity and improve performance. Leaders who use active listening discover the strengths of individuals and groups within their organization. Leaders who provide positive reinforcement and rewards, expect excellence, and remove barriers to employee involvement in the work process enable their employees to feel empowered, recognized and acknowledged as valuable. Leaders must base their responses on actual assessment, rather than preconceived ideas or biases. The four greatest motivators for employees are:

- **Autonomy**: Allowing people to use their ideas
- **Salary**: Providing adequate compensation for work done
- **Recognition**: Appreciating the efforts that employees put forth
- **Respect**: Listening to ideas.

There are three theories that leaders may consider when identifying additional ways to engage with and further understand what motivates their employees:

- **Expectancy theory** suggests that employees want to be sure that their effort correlates with their definition of success. Employees that follow this motivation system feel most connected when there is a clear performance rating system that allows them to monitor their progress and provides a clear path for outcomes.
- **Equity theory** suggests that employees are motivated when they feel the work environment is fair.
- **Procedural justice** suggests that employees are motivated by fairness related to procedures and processes. This means that employees want to be heard without bias and be able to provide input when important decisions are made.

An important aspect of motivating staff is understanding how to effectively promote change through proper communication and understanding amongst a team. Innovation is occurring rapidly within the industry and healthcare quality professionals are uniquely positioned to disseminate information and encourage team members as change occurs within organizations. The Institute for Healthcare Improvement (IHI) has a framework that provides guidance on how to approach spreading change in an organization quickly. This framework contains seven components for consideration:

- **Leadership** has a responsibility to ensure that any change aligns with long-term strategic goals. Key sponsors are identified and communication plans are established.
- **Setup for spread** means that infrastructure should be in place to target the ideal population, and a strategy for implementation should be developed.
- **Better ideas** describes the process of making the business case for an idea to get buy-in. Building the business case involves effectively communicating the value added by moving forward with a particular idea and gaining support within the organization to proceed.
- **Communication** describes establishing methods for spreading awareness and information about changes.
- **Social system** relates to having an understanding of the relationships amongst all parties involved in making a change.

- **Knowledge management** describes gathering data to determine whether the process change requires modification or if there is a better practice that can be implemented.
- **Measurement and feedback** involves developing a system to track whether the spread of change is occurring as anticipated.

Another framework aligned with motivating staff and leading change is **Rogers' diffusion of innovation model**. Rogers proposes two key points in this model:

- There are five **stages to embrace innovation**: knowledge, persuasion, decision, implementation, and confirmation.
- There are five **types of adopter categories** within a target population:
    - **Innovators** represent 2.5% of the population and are the first to want to try a change or innovation
    - **Early adopters** represent 13.5% of the population and embrace change. They do not need additional information to convince them to change.
    - **Early majority** represent 34% of the population and require proof that a change or innovation works prior to committing.
    - **Late majority** represent 34% of the population and are often skeptical of any change.
    - **Laggards** represent 16% of the population and are the hardest to encourage to change. These are often very traditional individuals that will require targeted strategies to encourage change.

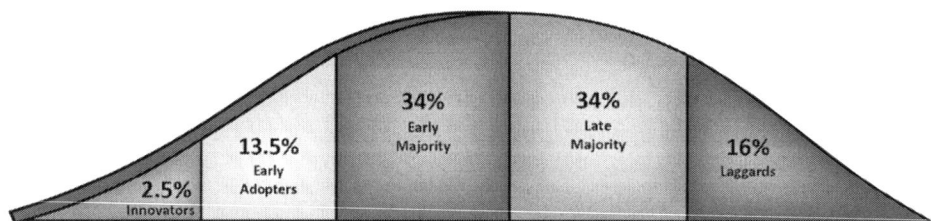

ORGANIZATIONAL CULTURE

Organizational culture comprises the attitudes, beliefs, and behaviors of those involved in the organization. The physical environment and the organizational structure strongly impact culture. Culture involves shared assumptions about behavior and working together in an organization. To facilitate change within an organization, the leader must understand its basic underlying values and change the organizational culture, along with changing processes and procedures.

Elements of culture include:

- **Values and norms** are the core beliefs and practices shared throughout the organization.
- **Symbols** are a representation of organizational culture and help spread aspects of company values. For example, an organization's logo is a symbol.
- **Language, slogans, and brands** communicate the identity of the organization.
- **Rituals and ceremonies** refer to events that reinforce culture.
- **Stories, legends, and myths** are narratives shared that demonstrate the organizational culture.
- **Heroes** are company role models who reinforce aspects of the organizational culture and lead by example.

The four basic **types of organizational cultures** are:

- **Stable learning cultures**, where people exercise skills and advance over time
- **Independent cultures**, in which people have valued skills that are easily transferable to other organizations
- **Group cultures**, in which there is strong identification and emphasis on seniority
- **Insecure cultures,** with frequent staff layoffs and reorganizations

To facilitate changes in the organizational culture, the leader must foster a commitment to excellence at all levels, create opportunities for involvement, and empower staff. Management must be flexible, encourage team building, and systems thinking across the organization.

CHANGE
FACILITATING CHANGE WITHIN THE HEALTHCARE SYSTEM

Facilitating change within a healthcare organization requires the creation of a common vision for care and begins with the organization creating teams to work collaboratively and focus on serving the customers. Achieving a common vision requires a true collaborative effort:

- Include all levels of staff across the organization, encompassing nursing and all other positions.
- Build consensus through discussions, in-service training, and team meetings, so diverse viewpoints converge.
- Value staff creativity and provide encouragement during the facilitation process.
- Post the common vision statement so it is accessible to all staff.
- Recognize that a common vision is an organic concept that evolves over time, requiring regular re-evaluation and changes as needed, so it continues to reflect the needs of the organization, patients, families, and staff.

When facilitating change within a healthcare organization, it is also important to appropriately assess the **limits of human performance** in being able to respond to change and the actual **capacity of the system** to handle change. Without consideration of these factors in development of a change initiative, there is a greater possibility of resistance from the systems that must make changes in order to achieve success.

LEWIN'S CHANGE MODEL

Force field analysis was designed by Kurt Lewin, a social psychologist, to analyze both the driving forces and the restraining forces for change:

- **Driving forces** instigate and promote change, such as leaders, incentives, and competition.
- **Restraining forces** resist change, such as poor attitudes, hostility, inadequate equipment, or insufficient funding.

For change to occur, the driving forces must be stronger than the restraining forces. It is easier to address and resolve restraining forces present within a team than to add additional driving forces.

Use this force field analysis diagram to discuss variables related to a proposed change in process:

- Write the proposed change in the center column.
- Brainstorm and list driving and restraining forces. Score the forces. (When driving and restraining forces are in balance, this is a state of equilibrium or the status quo.)
- Discuss the value of the proposed change.
- Develop a plan to diminish or eliminate restraining forces.

PALMER'S CHANGE MODEL

Palmer's change model focuses on seven elements required to shift an organization from its current state to its ideal state:

- Leading change
- Creating a shared need
- Shaping a vision
- Mobilizing commitment
- Monitoring progress
- Finishing the job
- Anchoring the change in systems and structure

In this change model, all seven elements are present within the transition from current state to ideal state. The first several elements focus on being able to successfully lead the change within the organization, while the remaining elements focus on being able to secure the change within the organization.

DEWEAVER AND GILLESPIE'S CHANGE MODEL

DeWeaver and Gillespie's change model focuses on understanding various stages of change and assessing which stage a team member aligns with to strategically plan next steps. There are 5 stages to take into consideration:

- The **awareness stage** occurs when an individual is cognizant of an upcoming change, but at this point has no bias regarding the impact the change will have on them.
- The **curiosity stage** occurs when an individual begins to inquire about a change. It is during this stage that emotions begin to arise, often due to concern regarding the change and potential negative impacts.
- The **visualization stage** occurs when an individual enters the initial stages of accepting the change. This includes asking questions to understand the implications of the change and gather information in order to prepare.
- The **learning stage** occurs when an individual participates in the change, actively implementing the change and providing feedback for improvement.
- The **use stage** occurs when an individual has fully incorporated the change and now has the experience to educate others on the change.

Of note, these stages are not linear. An individual may progress from the awareness stage directly to the learning stage, only to revert back to the curiosity stage after a particular experience.

Galpin's Change Model

Galpin's change model places emphasis on understanding human behavior and establishing structure for effective change management. The concept of change is broken into two components:

- Strategic
    - Stage 1: Establishing the need to change
    - Stage 2: Developing and disseminating a vision of change
    - Stage 3: Diagnosing/analyzing the current situation
    - Stage 4: Generating recommendations
    - Stage 5: Detailing recommendations
- Grassroots
    - Stage 6: Pilot-testing recommendations
    - Stage 7: Preparing recommendations for rollout
    - Stage 8: Rolling out changes
    - Stage 9: Measuring, reinforcing, and refining changes

Galpin suggests that, through this 9-step process and the intentional effort to consider more than the technical aspects of change, organizations are better positioned for success. An additional component of Galpin's change model includes consideration of how communication takes place during a change. Within the 9 stages of change, it is critical to consider the importance of building awareness (stages 1-2), communicating project status (stages 3-7), rolling out a communication plan (stage 8) and following up with staff (stage 9).

Kotter's Heart of Change Model

Kotter's heart of change model focuses on individuals intentionally integrating change into their belief system to create major change. Through a series of eight stages, organizations can shift from complacency to sustainable change:

- **Create a sense of urgency** through communicating the importance of the required change.
- **Build the right team** to coordinate and guide the process of change effectively.
- **Establish a vision** and the associated initiatives to communicate how goals will be achieved.
- **Get buy-in** to ensure all parties are committed to working towards the same goal.
- **Remove barriers** to empower action.
- **Create and recognize short-term wins**.
- **Sustain progress**.
- **Make change stick** through communicating the importance of maintaining changed behaviors for organizational success.

Through Kotter's process, organizations will avoid many of the barriers that prevent change efforts. Most initiatives will progress through all eight stages; however, it is not uncommon for multiple stages to occur simultaneously.

PROCHASKA'S TRANSTHEORETICAL CHANGE MODEL

Prochaska's transtheoretical change model, also known as the **stages of change** model, is designed to identify ways to implement change at an individual level through behavior. There are five stages:

- **Precontemplation** is the "not ready" phase – individuals in this phase have no intention of taking action within the next 6 months.
- **Contemplation** is the "getting ready" phase – individuals in this phase intend to take action within the next 6 months.
- **Preparation** is the "ready" phase when an individual has intention to act within the next month. There is typically a plan of action already in place.
- **Action** is the "making change" phase when an individual has demonstrated observable change within the last 6 months.
- **Maintenance** is the "keeping up change" phase when an individual has sustained change for at least 6 months.

BARRIERS TO SYSTEM CHANGE

Barriers to system change can arise at the individual, departmental, or administrative levels because of:

- **Identification with role rather than purpose**: People see themselves from the perspective of their role in the system (e.g., as a nurse or as a physician) and are not able to step outside their preconceived ideas to view situations holistically or to accept the roles of others. They may lack the ability to look at situations as human beings first and professionals second.
- **Feelings of victimization**: People may blame the organization or the leadership for personal shortcomings, or feel that there is nothing that they can do to improve or change situations. A feeling of victimization may permeate an institution to the point that meaningful communication cannot take place, and people are closed to change.
- **Relying on past experience**: New directions require new solutions, so being mired in the past or relying solely on past experience can prevent progress.
- **Autocratic views**: Autocrats feel that their perceptions and practices are the only ones that are acceptable, and often have a narrow focus, so that they cannot view the system as a whole but focus on short-term outcomes. They fail to see that there are many aspects to a problem, affecting many parts of the healthcare system.
- **Failure to adapt**: Change is difficult for many individuals and institutions, but the medical world is changing rapidly and this requires adaptability. Those who fail to adapt may feel threatened by changes and unsure of their ability to relearn new concepts, principles, and procedures.
- **Weak consensus**: Groups that arrive at an easy or weak consensus without delving into important issues may delude themselves into believing that they have solved problems, which remain fixed and are often ignored, rather than moving forward to resolution.

Dealing with Resistance to Organizational Change

Performance improvement processes cannot occur without organizational change, but **resistance to change** is common for many people who fear job loss or increased responsibilities. Staff may suffer from denial, lack understanding, or be frustrated by bureaucracy. The effective CPHQ anticipates resistance. Achieve cooperation with this approach:

- Be honest, informative, and tactful; give people thorough information about anticipated changes and how they will be affected, emphasizing positives.
- Be patient; allow people the time they need to contemplate changes and express anger or disagreement.
- Be empathetic; listen carefully to the concerns of others.
- Encourage participation; allow staff to propose methods of implementing change, so they feel a sense of ownership.
- Establish a climate in which all staff members are encouraged to identify the need for change on an ongoing basis.
- Present further ideas for change to management.

> **Review Video: Organizational Change Management Theories**
> Visit mometrix.com/academy and enter code: 404217

Crisis Management

Coordinating performance improvement involves crisis management preparation because the public is concerned about events that affect the quality of patient care. Consider terrorist acts, epidemics, natural disasters, financial malfeasance, public relations issues, and sentinel events when planning. Crisis management requires an organization-wide commitment to preventing crises. The two elements of crisis management are:

- **Preventive**, which includes establishing control barriers, conducting root cause analysis, direct observation and readiness activities, preparing contingency plans, and designing processes with failure mode and effects analysis (FMEA).
- **Reactive**, which includes root cause analysis of observed problems, determining long- and short-term effects, assigning staff to deal with issues, and looking for improvement opportunities.

Conflict Resolution

Conflict is an inevitable product of teamwork. The team leader assumes responsibility for conflict resolution and has a plan ready. Conflicts can be disruptive, or they can produce positive outcomes by opening dialogue and allowing team members to experience different perspectives. The best time for conflict resolution is when differences first emerge, before open conflict and hardened positions appear. Use active listening. Reassure those involved that their viewpoints are understood. Follow these steps for conflict resolution:

1. Allow both sides to present their opinions. Focus on opinions, rather than on individuals.
2. Encourage cooperation through negotiation and compromise.
3. Keep discussions on track and avoid heated arguments.
4. Evaluate the need for renegotiation, a formal resolution process, or third-party arbitration.
5. Use humor and empathy to defuse escalating tensions.
6. Summarize the issues. Outline key arguments.
7. Avoid forcing a resolution, if possible.

PROBLEM SOLVING

Problem solving in any medical context involves arriving at a hypothesis and then testing and assessing data to determine if the hypothesis holds true. When a problem arises, these steps help avoid a recurrence:

1. **Resolve** the immediate problem.
2. **Define** the larger issue by talking with the patient, his or her family, and staff to determine if the problem is related to a failure of communication or other issues, such as culture or religion.
3. **Collect data** by interviewing additional staff or reviewing documents, to gain a variety of perspectives.
4. **Identify important concepts** to determine if there are issues related to values or beliefs.
5. **Consider reasons for actions** to distinguish the motives and intentions of all parties, which underlie the problem.
6. **Decide** how to prevent a recurrence of the problem based on patient advocacy and moral agency; reach the best solution possible for the patient and family.

EIGHT DISCIPLINES OF PROBLEM SOLVING (8D)

The Eight Disciplines of Problem Solving (8D) were developed by the military and later refined by Ford Motor Company and Kepner-Tregoe. 8D helps teams to efficiently determine root causes of problems. 8D is used primarily in the industrial sector to improve product and process, but it also has direct applications to process improvement in healthcare. The disciplines are:

- Create and define an interdisciplinary team of experts with time and commitment to change. Establish roles within the team, needs, and guidelines. The team chooses their leader.
- Identify and describe the problem, including the scope and whether it is a common cause or special cause condition. Begin the process of identifying and gathering data.
- Take interim containment action (ICA, corrective actions) by insulating internal and external customers from problems and establishing criteria for decisions, while continuing to monitor results of the ICA.
- Identify and verify root causes and special cause conditions, using such methods as root-cause analysis, Five Whys, or Is–Is Not. Test each possible cause in accordance with the problem and data.
- Choose permanent corrective action (PCA). Establish criteria. List possible long-term solutions and prioritize them. Set up barrier controls to prevent the problem from recurring before committing to the action. Identify any negative side effects from the action and correct them.
- Implement PCA and remove ICA while conducting performance measures, documenting changes, and evaluating effectiveness.
- Perform evaluation to prevent recurrence. Modify procedures as necessary. Carry out formal processes to institute and communicate changes in action. Institute staff training as needed.
- Recognize the team members for their contributions and disband the team.

IS–IS NOT METHOD

Is–Is Not is a quality control method to identify root causes of problems and keep the team focused on the immediate problem.

- Create a table with a header above two columns. Write the problem at the top, in the header. Title one column "Is," and the other "Is Not."
- Ask who, what, where, when, why, and how in relation to the process. Do not focus on the people involved. Create a detailed description of the problem or event. When the problem or event is concretely identified, write it in the "Is" column.
- Ask what things could have caused the same problem, but did not. Evaluate similar processes in which the problem did not occur. When what the problem or event is not is identified, write a detailed description in the "Is Not" column.
- Compare the two columns of information. Determine what distinguishes them to help find potential causes.
- Identify changes that occurred, resulting in the problem, which leads to a root cause.

FIVE WHYS

The Five Whys is a method of finding root causes and solving problems designed by Taiichi Ohno of Toyota, in Japan. This process requires a pre-trained, knowledgeable team, who asks "why" in a sequential manner, to narrow the focus and arrive at consensus about the cause of an event. The steps are:

- Outline the process in detail and describe each event in the sequence of events.
- Ask "why" questions about each step in the sequence of events to try to determine cause. For example:
    - Q: Why did the patient return to the Emergency Department?
    - A: Because the doctor initially failed to order an x-ray of the patient's injured hand.
    - Q: Why did the doctor fail to order an x-ray of the patient's injured hand?
    - A: Because the Radiology Department was understaffed and there was a two-hour delay to obtain x-rays.
- Reach a consensus and propose solutions to improve performance.

Performance Improvement Methods

JURAN QUALITY PLANNING PROCESS

The Juran quality planning process is a systematic approach to the development of action plans and can be used for strategic plans, quality design, patient safety programs, clinical standards, benchmarking, development of performance measures, and parts of process improvement. It may be used to design new processes or to modify or redesign previously existing processes:

- **Establish the project**: Prioritize, establish teams, and write goals.
- **Identify customers**: Completely assess the internal and external customers and their needs.
- **Design or redesign the implementation process**: Describe the current process. Perform a literature review. Identify benchmarks and best practices. Assess customer needs, in light of the latest information available.
- **Evaluate needs**: This includes evaluating training, implementation costs (in terms of time, staff, and money), resource needs, and expected outcomes.

PDCA PERFORMANCE IMPROVEMENT MODEL

Plan-Do-Check-Act (PDCA or Shewhart cycle) is a method of continuous quality improvement. PDCA is simple and understandable; however, it may be difficult to maintain this cycle consistently because of lack of focus and commitment. PDCA is more suited to solving specific problems, rather than organization-wide problems. The model starts with the Plan phase and works in a continuous cycle. Details of each phase are included below:

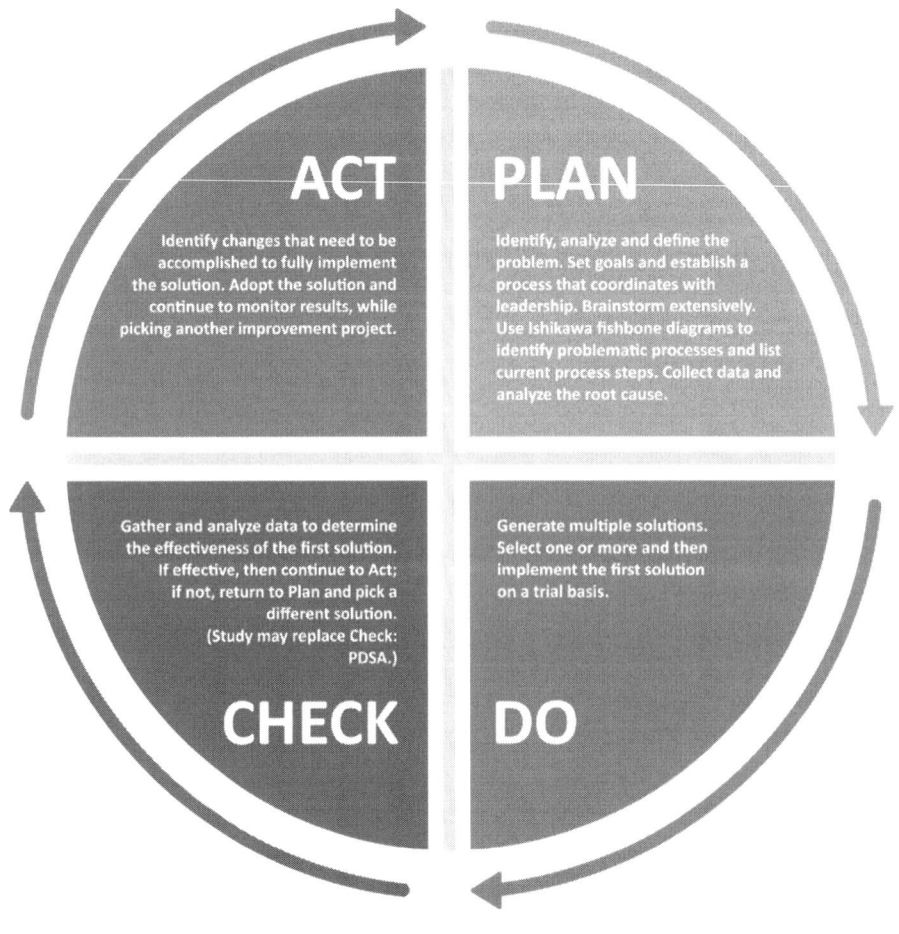

FOCUS Performance Improvement Model

Find, organize, clarify, uncover, and start (FOCUS) is a performance improvement model that is focused on process improvement:

- **Find**: Identify a problem by looking at the organization and attempting to determine what isn't working well or what is wrong.
- **Organize**: Identify the people who understand the problem or process and create a team to work on improving performance.
- **Clarify**: Utilize brainstorming techniques, such as Ishikawa fishbone diagrams, to determine what is involved in solving the problem.
- **Uncover**: Analyze the situation to determine the reason the problem has arisen or why a process is unsuccessful.
- **Start**: Determine where to begin the change process.

FOCUS, by itself, is an incomplete process and is primarily used as a means to identify a problem, rather than a means to find the solution. FOCUS is usually combined with PDCA (FOCUS-PDCA), so it becomes a 9-step process. Beginning with FOCUS refines the problem, resulting in better outcomes.

Accelerated Rapid-Cycle Change Model

The accelerated rapid-cycle change approach is a response to rapid changes in healthcare delivery and radical re-engineering. Rapid cycle improvement has the foundation of PDCA, but relies on incremental improvements to be able to quickly assess and determine next steps. There are four areas of concern:

- **Models for rapid-cycle change**: The goal is doubling or tripling the rate of quality improvement by modifying and accelerating traditional methods. Teams focus on generating and testing solutions, rather than analysis.
- **Pre-work**: Assigned personnel prepare problem statements, graphic demonstrations of data, flowcharts, and a literature review. Team members are identified.
- **Team creation**: Rapid action teams (RATs, or rapid acceleration, or rapid achievement) are created to facilitate quick change.
- **Team meetings** and **work flow** are done over the course of 6 weeks:
    - Week 1: Review information. Clarify quality improvement opportunities. Identify key customers, waste, and benchmarks.
    - Week 2: Review customer requirements. Perform a cost/benefit analysis of the solution with test data.
    - Week 3: Complete the solution's design. Plan its implementation. Conduct pilot tests.
    - Weeks 4-5: Test, train, analyze, and make changes as needed.
    - Week 6: Implement the solution.

Xerox 10-Step Benchmarking Model

Benchmarking is an ongoing process of measuring practice, service, or product results against their competitors' or industry standards. **Xerox Corporation** developed the **10-step benchmarking model**. The CPHQ needs to know how efficient others' processes are and search their data for ways to improve the processes. There are four phases in benchmarking: **Planning**, **analysis**, **integration**, and **action**. The 10 steps are:

1. Identify the benchmark targets.
2. Identify similar organizations with which to compare data.
3. Determine and initiate methods of data collection.
4. Evaluate current performance level and deficits.
5. Project a vision of future performance.
6. Communicate findings and reach a group agreement.
7. Recommend changes, based on benchmarking data.
8. Develop specific action plans for objectives.
9. Implement actions and adjust them as necessary, based on monitoring of the process.
10. Update benchmarks based on the latest data.

This basic benchmarking model is often modified. It can be shortened to 7 steps, or extended to 11 steps, depending on the needs of the organization. Benchmarking is often used to improve cash flow, as healthcare becomes more competitive, and to compare infection rates.

Ernst and Young's 7-Step IMPROVE Model

The Ernst and Young 7-step IMPROVE model is a simplified model that is effective for teams who are already experienced with quality improvement processes and data collection. The basic steps for the IMPROVE model are:

- **Identify**: Select a problem and evaluate current performance.
- **Measure**: Determine its impact on internal and external customers through evaluation of data.
- **Prioritize**: Identify all possible causes for the problem and prioritize them.
- **Research**: Assess and evaluate the problem, including a root cause analysis.
- **Outline**: Determine all possible solutions to the problem and develop an action plan to implement appropriate solutions.
- **Validate**: Establish a monitoring system after implementation to validate the effectiveness of a solution.
- **Execute**: Continue to fully implement the solutions and standardize them, while continuing to monitor efficiency.

ORGANIZATIONAL DYNAMICS FADE CYCLE PERFORMANCE IMPROVEMENT MODEL

Organizational Dynamics, a consulting firm, developed a four-phase **FADE performance cycle for quality improvement.** The FADE model uses outputs and inputs. The output from one phase serves as the input for the next. The phases are as follows:

1. **Focus**: Hold brainstorming sessions to create a list of problems. Select one problem. Define the problem, analyze its impact completely, and generate a problem statement (output).
2. **Analyze**: Collect baseline data, identify patterns, and gather general information about factors that influence the problem or outcomes. Make charts and diagrams (output), such as Pareto, fishbones, and flowcharts.
3. **Develop**: Generate a list of possible solutions and choose one solution. Create an action plan for implementation (output).
4. **Execute**: Develop support and commitment for the proposed solution through presentations. Put the plan into effect (output). Monitor the plan's impact to ensure that the plan is effective.

JURAN QUALITY IMPROVEMENT PROCESS (QIP) MODEL

Joseph Juran's Quality Improvement Process (QIP) is a three-step model, focusing on quality control. QIP is based on quality planning, control, and improvement. The steps to the QIP are:

1. **Define the problem**: Organize the project by listing and prioritizing problems, and identifying a team.
2. **Analyze the problem**: Analyze the problems and then formulate theories related to their root cause. Test theories.
3. **Implement solutions**: Consider various alternative solutions. Design and implement specific solutions and controls. Address institutional resistance to change. As causes of problems are identified, remediate them, and processes should improve.

LEAN PERFORMANCE IMPROVEMENT MODEL

Lean is the process of creating value for customers through the elimination of waste. Removing steps that do not create value ensures productivity. While the concept of lean originated in the manufacturing industry, many other industries, such as healthcare, have adopted lean principles to improve outcomes for customers. Since removing waste is a critical step prior to achieving optimal performance, lean is often practiced in organizations prior to introducing Six Sigma. Within lean, there are eight types of waste to consider:

- **Transportation waste** is waste that occurs when materials are moved farther or more frequently than is necessary.
- **Inventory waste** is waste resulting from an excess of stored work-in-progress.
- **Motion waste** is energy expended by the unnecessary physical movement of workers.
- **Waiting waste** is the time lost while waiting until the next step in the process can occur.
- **Overproduction waste** is waste from producing more goods than customers will use.
- **Overprocessing waste** occurs when more work is being done than is required to meet established standards.
- **Defects waste** is waste resulting from errors or subpar work.
- **Unused talent waste** occurs when a worker has more valuable skills than are being used.

Six Sigma Performance Improvement Model

Six Sigma is a performance improvement model developed by Motorola to improve its business practices and increase its profits. The Six Sigma model has been adapted to many types of businesses, including healthcare. Six Sigma is a data-driven performance model that aims to eliminate "defects" in processes that involve products or services. The goal is to achieve Six Sigma, meaning no more than 3.4 defects in every 1 million opportunities. The focus is on continuous improvement, with the customer's perception as key, so that the customer defines what is critical to quality (CTQ). Two different types of improvement projects may be employed: DMAIC (define, measure, analyze, improve, control) for existing processes or products that need improvement and DMADV (define, measure, analyze, design, verify) for development of new, high-quality processes or products. Both DMAIC and DMADV utilize trained personnel to execute the plans. Six Sigma personnel have martial arts titles:

- **Yellow belts** have basic knowledge regarding Six Sigma and participate in improvement projects as team members, receiving guidance from those leading the initiative.
- **Green belts** and **black belts** both execute programs; however, black belts have additional training and often oversee projects led by green belts, ensuring accuracy in data collection and communication with those involved in the initiative.
- **Master black belts** supervise programs through development of metrics, providing strategic insight and training.

DMAIC Type of Six Sigma Performance Improvement Project

The first project type for Six Sigma is **DMAIC** (define, measure, analyze, improve, control), which is used when existing healthcare processes or products need quality improvement:

- **Define** the problem, customer, stakeholders, and key metrics in order to communicate why the quality improvement initiative is taking place. Establish the project scope and deadlines to ensure success. Use a project charter to formally outline components of the initiative and track progress.
- **Measure** input, process, and output. Collect baseline data. Perform a cost analysis. Calculate the sigma rating. Use a control chart to track how the process is changing over time.
- **Analyze** root or other causes of current defects. Use data to confirm analysis. Uncover steps in processes that are counterproductive. Utilize tools such as a Fishbone diagram or value stream map to determine where to focus efforts.
- **Improve** by creating potential solutions. Develop and pilot plans. Measure the results. Determine the cost savings and other benefits to customers.
- **Control** the work processes by standardizing them. Monitor the system by linking performance measures to a balanced scorecard. Create processes for updating procedures, disseminating reports, and recommending future processes.

LEAN SIX SIGMA PERFORMANCE IMPROVEMENT MODEL

Lean Six Sigma is a performance improvement model that combines Six Sigma with concepts of Lean thinking by focusing process improvement on strategic goals, rather than specific projects. A Lean Six Sigma program is driven by strong senior leadership, who outline long-term goals and strategies to employees. Physicians are an important part of the Lean Six Sigma process in the healthcare context and must be included and engaged. The basis of Lean Six Sigma is to reduce errors and waste within the organization through continuous learning and rapid change.

- **Long-term goals** with strategies in place for 1- to 3-year periods
- **Performance improvement** as the underlying belief system
- **Cost reduction** through quality increase, supported by statistics evaluating the cost of inefficiency
- **Incorporation of improvement methodology**, such as DMAIC, PDCA, or other methods

Quality Tools and Techniques

Lean Six Sigma Tools

Common tools used by healthcare quality professionals during Lean Six Sigma initiatives include:

- **Value Stream Mapping** (VSM) is a performance improvement tool that visually depicts the steps of a process to identify priorities from a customer perspective. It is most often used in lean performance improvement activities, as it is a tool that identifies areas of waste that can be removed.
- **6S** is a tool designed to eliminate waste and increase productivity. It is best used when order needs to be established in the workplace. 6S consists of Sort, Set in Order, Shine, Safety, Standardize and Sustain. All components together achieve workplace safety.
- A **spaghetti diagram** is a visualization of the flow of a process and traces the steps from start to finish. This tool is used to gain an understanding of redundancies in a process.
- **SIPOC** stands for Suppliers, Input, Process, Output, Customer. SIPOC is a process management tool that helps identify critical components of a process. This tool is used to develop an understanding of the source of materials or product, the resources needed and how value is created for the customer.

National and International Quality Models

There is an increasing need for both national and international excellence/quality models, so that best practices and standardizations can be shared. Existing models include:

- **Joint Commission Standards for Improvement of Organizational Performance**, where voluntary compliance leads to accreditation.
- The **National Committee for Quality Assurance (NCQA)** management improvement process.
- **Baldrige Award Criteria for Process Management and Results**, an evaluation process providing excellent performance assessment.
- **International Standards Organization (ISO)** standard for quality management (9001:2000), which requires a strategic approach to process improvement through quality planning and supportive data.
- **United States Federal Quality Improvement Programs,** which help organizations remain in compliance with these complex federal mandates regarding Medicare through the following:
  - Healthcare Quality Improvement Program (HCQIP)
  - Quality Improvement Organization (QIO) projects
  - Quality Improvement System for Managed Care (QISMC)

Healthcare facilities participate in these models to obtain accreditation, comply with Medicare or other federal program regulations, gain feedback, or gain prestige.

Quality Improvement Projects

The steps the CPHQ must take for coordination of quality improvement projects are as follows:

1. Secure support, resources, and approval from the governing board and key administrative and professional leaders, building support and commitment.
2. Build relationships among staff to facilitate change.
3. Assess the needs of the organization, the climate for change, and the extent of support and resistance in the organization.

4. Produce an internal action plan that describes problems that need resolution, development needs, process steps to be completed, responsible staff, and a timeline for completion of tasks.
5. Delineate resource needs, including staffing and training, with a detailed budget outlining the statistical, clerical, and technical needs.
6. Clarify roles and responsibilities organization-wide.
7. Educate staff regarding the mission, vision, values, philosophy of quality management, techniques and tools, benefits, and accreditation and regulatory needs.

Building effectiveness into quality improvement projects requires an ongoing commitment at all levels of the organization. The CPHQ oversees the following elements:

- Clearly identify leadership roles at all levels in writing.
- Consistently use a common quality language, such as quality management (QM), continuous quality management (CQM), and total quality management (TQM).
- Simplify the accountability structure and eliminate redundancy, determining which bodies have ultimate responsibility for decisions and prioritizing, such as a Quality Council.
- Create a flow chart that outlines the quality improvement structure.
- Align organization policies, mission, vision statements, and strategic goals to quality improvement goals.
- Identify organizational functions, including patient care.
- Outline the methodology for performance improvement.
- Establish a structure for periodic reporting and summaries.
- Create interdisciplinary teams.
- Write an implementation plan for organization-wide quality improvement.
- Identify education needs and provide training for teams and leaders.

EVENTS AND CAUSAL FACTORS CHART

The events and causal factors analysis (E&CF) chart is a combination of the flow chart and affinity diagram. E&CF lists the sequential steps in a process or occurrence and the conditions affecting each step. E&CF is useful in root cause analysis and to analyze best practices. The steps for E&CF are as follows:

1. List the name of the process or occurrence in a box on the right (as in a flow chart).
2. List the steps in the process in boxes from right to left (as in a cause-effect diagram), linked with arrows pointing to the process box on the right.
3. Under each event box, place an arrow pointing downward and list all possible factors that contributed to the occurrence at that step through repeatedly asking "Why?" (as in an affinity diagram).
4. Discuss and reach group consensus about root causes to determine actions for performance improvement or (if used to analyze best practices) to ensure a process can be replicated.

Storyboards

A storyboard is a visual representation of the actions of a team, including data analysis and decisions, during the performance improvement process. It is usually done on a firm poster board, around 3-4 feet square. A storyboard looks somewhat like a giant flow chart, with arrows or lines connecting one piece of information to the next. A storyboard includes a wide variety of information, including the following:

- Charts
- Diagrams
- Pictures
- Text
- Illustrations
- Statistics

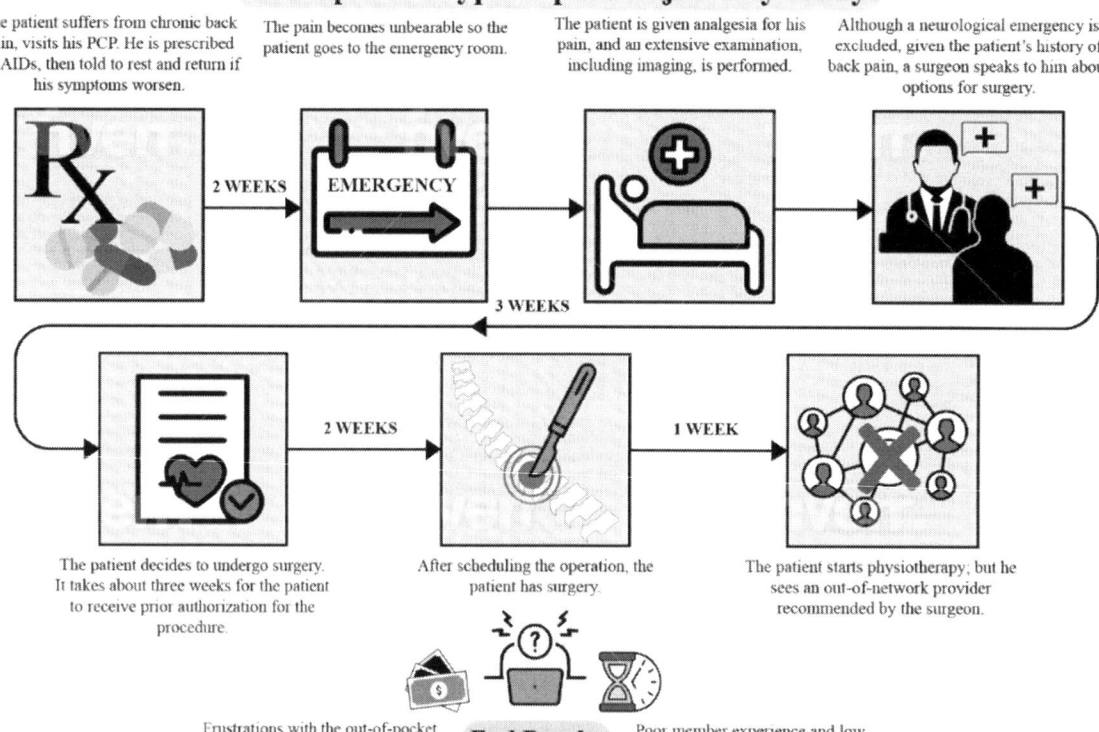

Because the storyboard is meant to provide easy access to information about team activities, keep text minimal.

Gantt Charts

A Gantt chart is a bar chart with a horizontal time scale used to:

- Develop improvement projects
- Manage schedules
- Estimate time needed to complete tasks

It is a visual representation of the beginning and end time points when different steps in a process should be completed. Gantt charts are available in project management software programs, Excel, and SmartDraw. Create a Gantt chart after initial brainstorming, to outline a timeline and action plans:

- List the name of the process in the header.
- Create a horizontal chart with the timeline of days, weeks, or months (as appropriate for the process) across the top.
- List tasks vertically on the left of the chart.
- Draw horizontal lines or bars from the expected beginning point to the expected end point for each task. Color-code task bars to indicate which individual or team is responsible for completing the task.

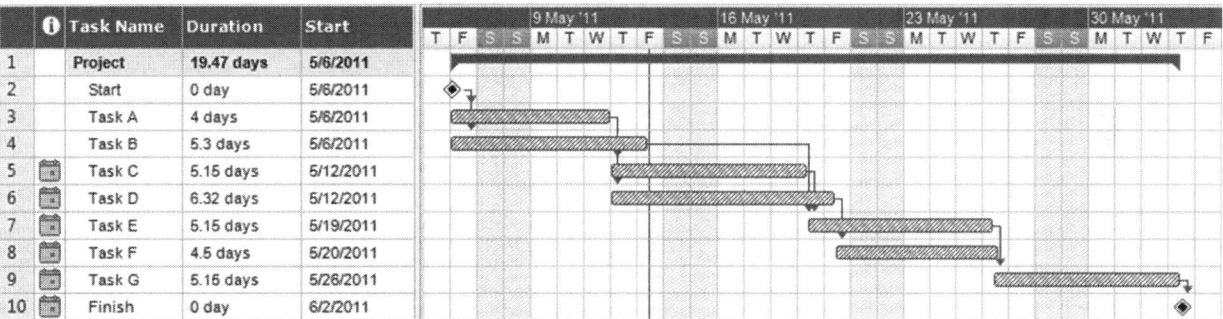

Task Lists

A task list is a simple but essential tool for organizing and developing plans. It assigns responsibility and helps individuals and teams stay within a scheduled time frame:

- Brainstorm to identify and discuss necessary tasks or steps in a process.
- Create a complete master list of tasks and steps.
- Assign responsibility for each task and step to an individual team member.
- Provide a timeframe during which the task or step must be completed.
- Create a task list in chart form, with 4 columns:
    - (Left) Task or step
    - (2nd) Individual responsible for completing task or step
    - (3rd) Due date for completion
    - (Right) Date the task or step is completed
- Update the list as tasks are completed. Share the revised task list with team members, so they can evaluate progress and identify tasks that have not been completed.

RASCI CHART

A RASCI chart, also known as a RASCI matrix, is a tool utilized by teams to clearly establish roles and responsibilities as a project or initiative progresses. RASCI charts encourage effective project management by assigning responsibility to avoid delays, miscommunication, or poor decision-making that often occurs without clear delineation of responsibilities. RASCI charts list out all of the tasks a project is expected to comprise, and for each task, team members are assigned responsibility under 5 categories:

- **Responsible**: Often referred to as the doer, this is the individual responsible for completing the assigned task. Every task must have one responsible individual.
- **Accountable**: This individual is accountable for the outcome of the task. It may or may not be the same individual who is responsible for carrying out the task. Every task must have one accountable individual.
- **Supportive**: This individual is a helper who assists the person who is responsible for the task. There may be more than one supportive individual assigned to a task or there may be none.
- **Consulted**: This is an individual within the project team that serves as a resource for the responsible individual and is consulted when expertise is needed or a decision requiring highly technical understanding needs to be made. There may be more than one consulted individual assigned to a task or there may be none.
- **Informed**: This individual must be informed of how a task is progressing at regular intervals. There may be more than one informed individual assigned to a task or there may be none.

DELPHI TECHNIQUE

The Delphi technique is a method of consensus-building that operates with the idea that, over time and with guidance, people will compromise and move toward similar opinions. This technique can be used to manipulate people's opinions through a series of methods such as brainstorming, multivoting, and nominal group technique. There are two different Delphi methods:

- **Method I**: A facilitator leads the group. Each member expresses an opinion, and then the facilitator challenges or questions these opinions, sometimes intimidating people into changing their positions, and other times facilitating a better exchange of ideas.
- **Method II**: A questionnaire or listing of options is given to each member so he/she can express an anonymous opinion (before, during, or after meetings). A facilitator or team leader then revises the questionnaire or listing of options, based on the responses, and circulates it again until consensus is reached. Discussion to review results takes place at team meetings.

Monitoring Timeliness

MONITORING PROJECT TIMELINESS AND DELIVERABLES

The measuring and monitoring of a project are ongoing procedures that evaluate progress toward objectives and indicate any deviations so that corrections can be made. Activities on the timeline should be assessed to determine if they are on schedule, ahead of schedule, or behind schedule. Risks should be assessed and managed. Changes should be assessed through integrated change control and all change requests documented as well as their approval or rejection. Quality control measurements should be carried out and any defects noted and corrected. Performance of team members should be monitored. Any changes in the scope of a project should be noted and the project plan updated. Performance reports should be completed as scheduled and disseminated to the proper individuals or agencies. A Gantt chart, which is a bar chart with a horizontal time scale that shows the start and finish dates for different steps in a process, may be used to develop and manage the timeline.

MONITORING CONSULTANTS

Many organizations hire consultants to facilitate or lead teams or to provide specific services for performance improvement. The CPHQ selects a consultant based on networking, recommendations, advertising, references, telephone interviews, presentations, personal interviews, and proposals. The CPHQ must select the correct consultant, to ensure that:

- Quality and patient safety are not compromised.
- The goals, needs, and budget of the project are met.

The duties of the CPHQ are to:

- Make a clear, itemized list of goals for the project.
- Provide an organizational chart to the consultant, clearly defining the lines of authority in relationship to the consultant.
- Create an itemized job description for the consultant.
- Specify time frames and deadlines in the consulting contract.
- Include confidentiality agreements and specific work requirements in the contract.

Once the consultant is hired, the CPHQ supervises the consultant's activities, to ensure that the consultant adheres to the job description and provides valued service to the organization.

Evaluating Effectiveness

DEMONSTRATING THE FINANCIAL BENEFITS OF A QUALITY PROGRAM

A quality performance improvement plan should not only improve functions (including patient care) but must show a **financial benefit** to the organization if it is to gain support of the governing board. Complete a cost-benefit analysis to demonstrate potential savings or income for each aspect of the action plan. For example, if bar coding will be used to decrease medication errors, thereby reducing complications and shortening hospital stay, then potential savings exist. Provide specific, measurable goals in the improvement plan to facilitate calculation of financial benefits. As the plan is implemented, include a financial benefit section in the monthly written report, because this provides tangible evidence of the plan's success. Summarize the financial benefits in graphs and charts, because a visual demonstration is a more effective way to communicate than text alone.

EVALUATING PERFORMANCE IMPROVEMENT MODELS

A number of different performance improvement models have been developed over the years. Evaluating and applying these models are part of strategic management and quality healthcare. Some medical organizations use a single approach, but many combine models in various ways in order to meet their specific needs. Those in leadership roles must understand how these models can facilitate change, so that they choose elements that are appropriate for the needs of their organization and those who will work with the model. All the various models share some elements:

- The models focus on **continuous improvement** and are planned, systematic, collaborative, and applicable to the entire organization.
- They all focus on identifying problems, collecting data, assessing current performance, instituting actions for change, assessing changes, team development, and use of data.
- In order for any model or eclectic elements from different models to be effective, there must be **cooperation** and **consensus** across the organization.

EVALUATION OF TEAM PERFORMANCE THROUGH PERFORMANCE MEASURES

Evaluation of team performance is a necessary part of performance improvement because of the need for efficient and effective teamwork. Teams are evaluated in three areas of performance:

- **Completion of assigned tasks**: This includes adhering to timelines, completing the task properly, and producing reports as required.
- **Ability of the group to work together and reach consensus**: A team must meet regularly, work effectively, and arrive at decisions with minimal conflict.
- **Effectiveness of the individual team members**: Team members must assume responsibility for completing their parts of tasks and cooperate with others in the group.

Consider each of these elements when developing performance measures for each step in a process to determine if the group is effective.

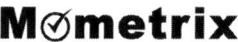

POOR TEAM PERFORMANCE INDICATORS

When analyzing data for evaluation of team performance, here are some indicators of poor performance:

- **Poor communication**: Communication is uneven. Team members don't listen to others or express opinions in a positive manner, and personality conflicts arise.
- **Poor problem solving**: Root cause analysis is not systematic or logical, so problems remain unresolved.
- **Lack of clarity**: Team members are unsure of their roles or responsibilities in the team or how the teamwork relates to strategic goals of the organization.
- **Inadequate management of timelines and deadlines**: Meetings are delayed or cancelled, projects are not completed on time, and reports are delayed.
- **Poor leadership**: The leader has no clear role and does not help the team to stay focused on tasks. Team members do not respect the leader.
- **Lack of interest and skills**: Team members do not want to participate, have personal problems, or lack necessary training, skills, or expertise to complete tasks.

Population Health and Care Transitions

Population Health

HEALTH STATUS OF A POPULATION

The health of a population is affected by social, environmental, and political factors that can influence health outcomes for a particular group. To determine the health status of a population, metrics such as life expectancy, mortality rates, and the prevalence or incidence of chronic conditions in specific populations need to be measured. These metrics can be obtained through various methods, such as targeted surveys, electronic health records, focus groups, town halls, or interviews with stakeholders. The data collected should include details that identify the factors that directly contribute to population health. These factors may include behavioral, environmental, and social determinants such as employment status, food security, social support, housing conditions, and other living conditions.

STRATEGIES USED TO IMPROVE INITIATIVES

The goal of population health management is to improve health outcomes and quality of care for groups of individuals while simultaneously containing costs. To achieve this goal, healthcare organizations need to focus on utilizing data analytics and payment models effectively. Addressing population health management requires access to both internal and external data sources and a thorough understanding of these data to support decision-making. This includes incorporating both clinical and nonclinical data to gain a comprehensive understanding of the population and drive strategic plans. Healthcare organizations should also have incentive systems in place to promote population health management strategies. For instance, value-based care initiatives incentivize providers and healthcare delivery systems for meeting specific quality, safety, and outcome targets for defined populations. By developing a focused plan that considers the data and current payment models, organizations can position themselves to perform well while also improving the health of the populations they serve.

DISEASE MANAGEMENT SOLUTIONS

The goal of disease management is to promote self-management of chronic conditions, such as diabetes or hypertension, through patient education. Effective disease management helps to reduce symptoms associated with chronic illnesses and prevent exacerbations that may lead to hospitalization. Healthcare organizations can incorporate disease management into their strategic goals by partnering with community organizations to promote prevention of chronic illness. For example, a healthcare organization may collaborate with a local food bank to ensure healthy food choices are available to community members. Disease management can also be integrated into strategic goals through the collaboration of multidisciplinary teams. By involving different specialties, disease management can be approached in a comprehensive and effective manner, improving patient outcomes and reducing costs for the healthcare system.

DISEASE MANAGEMENT PROGRAMS

An effective disease management program can address social determinants of health by focusing on the factors that contribute to chronic illness. Many chronic conditions are linked to environmental, cultural, and behavioral factors that people are exposed to during their upbringing. By taking these factors into consideration, a disease management program can initiate a comprehensive approach to positively impact individuals' overall health. For example, a disease management program can address access to healthcare, housing, food insecurity, and literacy.

Access to healthcare ensures that individuals have the resources and knowledge regarding healthcare available and are able to use them appropriately. Consistent access to safe housing and healthy food choices ensures that individuals can make better choices that lead to a healthier lifestyle. It also allows them to focus on their health rather than on survival concerns related to a lack of basic resources. Providing resources that enhance literacy ensures that individuals understand their chronic conditions and can make informed decisions about their health, leading to effective long-term self-management of their condition.

Supporting Health Equity

Health equity means ensuring that everyone has an equal opportunity to achieve their highest level of health. Achieving health equity requires addressing the barriers that prevent vulnerable populations from reaching their health goals. This may involve tackling social and economic barriers, such as modifying structural impediments, identifying institutional or systemic racism that may be preventing access to healthcare, or developing programs to reduce poverty and improve economic stability for marginalized groups.

Healthcare organizations can make a direct impact on health equity by partnering with community organizations that focus on improving health equity in their communities. For example, healthcare organizations can support after-school programs that assist at-risk children with homework. Healthcare organizations can also support health equity by identifying social determinants of health that are affecting their patient population. For instance, if a healthcare organization reviews data and identifies that a particular subset of patients is struggling with medication adherence due to financial strain, they may develop a partnership to participate in the 340B Drug Pricing Program to ensure that patients have access to affordable medication needed to manage their chronic conditions.

Addressing Health Disparities

Healthcare disparities refer to the differences in access and availability of healthcare services that result in unequal disease burden in disadvantaged groups. These disparities can be addressed by healthcare organizations through proper education and training to develop cultural competency, enabling providers and healthcare staff to intervene where necessary to break the cycle of health inequity. Additionally, healthcare organizations can strategically open locations in underserved areas to provide access to care and become involved in the local community to bring about change. For instance, healthcare organizations can organize events that promote health literacy among disadvantaged groups and provide resources through partnerships with community organizations. By identifying opportunities to address healthcare disparities, healthcare organizations can incorporate their findings into initiatives through the development of targeted goals to address health equity.

For example, a healthcare organization that partners with community organizations to provide care to the underinsured and uninsured may have identified an opportunity for improving health literacy in the population. As these data are brought to the attention of leadership, goals can be established internally to develop programs to assess and address health literacy in the patient population and the larger community.

Using Data to Drive and Monitor Improvement Efforts

Healthcare organizations can improve population health by using data to make informed decisions that positively impact the well-being of specific patient populations in real time. However, data can be siloed within organizations, making it challenging to come to comprehensive conclusions.

Healthcare quality professionals should develop skills to effectively analyze big data to support the development of actionable insights that bring awareness to the needs of a population.

Data that drive improvement efforts and provide insight into population health initiatives include both structured and unstructured data such as electronic health record data, patient-generated health data, and medication adherence data. Electronic health record data can provide details about claims, encounters, and social determinants of health, giving insight into a patient's health status and potential barriers to self-management of chronic conditions. Patient-generated health data can include information directly supplied by patients and/or their family through surveys or assessments, empowering patients to become active in their own healthcare.

Healthcare organizations can also capture social determinants of health through surveys and assessments to inform care teams about factors affecting an individual's health, such as unemployment or homelessness. By analyzing these data sources, healthcare organizations can identify areas for improvement and develop targeted interventions to improve the health of specific patient populations in real time.

Targeted Initiatives

Healthcare organizations can address social determinants of health by developing targeted initiatives that focus on developing awareness, advocacy, and alignment. Awareness involves identifying the specific needs of the population of interest. This can be done through patient surveys and assessments, or through focus groups conducted by culturally competent staff. The results of the research should support advocacy for additional resources or the development of partnerships that promote social change.

Alignment is achieved by identifying existing connections within the organization or among the organization and community partners. When solidified, these connections can address equity-oriented healthcare services. For example, a healthcare quality professional may identify data from patient experience surveys that indicate patients at the clinic have had trouble attending appointments due to a lack of transportation. The healthcare quality professional can use this data to support the request for bus fare for identified patient populations to improve healthcare outcomes and decrease the no-show rate. After the request is approved, the healthcare quality professional can align with the clinic's internal case management team to inform them of the new resource available. The professional can also develop a partnership with community organizations that provide medical transportation to ensure alignment.

Providing Outcome-Based, Cost-Effective Care

Outcome-based, cost-effective care integrates delivery of care with supporting data. It uses different approaches for cost-containment and quality improvement strategies. It is based on identification of a problem, collection of data (evidence), evaluation, integration of both data and patient needs to deliver patient care, and re-evaluation of the process. Evidence-based care requires a process of change in the healthcare system:

- Resources for staff, including guidelines, journals, and established protocols.
- A mission statement and goals that support evidence-based care.
- Staff input and dialog through in-service training, meetings, team building, mentoring, teaching, and role modeling.
- Allocation of resources and staff to gather and interpret data, assessing outcomes.

- Use of randomized controlled trials (RCTs) to determine which approaches are best combined with systematic research and review.
- Retaining an individual assessment to determine if data apply to the unique circumstances of each patient.

IMPACT OF QUALITY INITIATIVES ON REIMBURSEMENT

INDUSTRY TRANSITION

As the industry continues to transition from fee-for-service to value-based care, healthcare quality professionals play an integral role in ensuring healthcare delivery systems are well equipped to effectively operate under alternative reimbursement models. Healthcare has traditionally operated under a **fee-for-service (FFS) model**, where physicians and other healthcare providers are paid based on the number of services, treatments, and procedures provided to patients. This model encourages healthcare providers to increase utilization without considering whether an equally effective and lower cost alternative exists. As a result, over time, the fee-for-service model has created significant waste within the system, which has contributed to increasing healthcare costs for both patients and healthcare delivery systems. **Value-based care** has been introduced to alleviate the financial burden caused by the fee-for-service model and reform how health care is delivered and paid for by placing the focus for reimbursement on patient outcomes. Value-based care takes a qualitative approach and incentivizes providers based on outcomes that ensure patient care is safe, effective, timely, efficient, equitable, and patient-centered. By placing the focus on these six domains, healthcare continuously inches closer towards achieving the quadruple aim – better care for individuals, improving the health of populations, lowering costs, enhanced provider experience.

ALTERNATIVE PAYMENT MODELS

The goal of the Affordable Care Act (ACA) was to transform the healthcare industry through rewarding providers for quality of care. Several different payment models, called **alternative payment models (APMs)**, were introduced by the ACA. APMs provide additional incentives to providers that meet metrics related to quality of care. The main goal remains unchanged: provide better quality of care and patient outcomes without an increase in spending. There are many different types of APMs, including the following:

- **Episode of care/bundled payments** provides a lump sum for all services that are related to a condition or disease. For example, if a patient has open heart surgery, the physician, anesthesiologist, hospital, and other providers involved would be collectively reimbursed rather than individually. The reimbursement for an episode of care is based on historical cost for the service.
- **Capitation** reimburses providers a fixed amount for a period of time to cover all services for a particular population.
- **Pay for performance (P4P)** is a term used to describe programs that provide a payment in addition to traditional FFS payment for meeting specific quality goals. There are typically four types of measures in these programs: performance, outcome, patient experience, and structure/technology.
- **Shared savings and risk** provides an incentive for remaining under a pre-established spending target while being paid via FFS. If a provider spends above the pre-established spending target, that money serves as a penalty or "risk" required to be paid back. Examples of shared savings are applicable to accountable care organizations (ACOs). In an ACO, a group of providers voluntarily come together to provide care to a population and contain cost through preventive care.

Care Transitions

IDENTIFYING OPPORTUNITIES FOR IMPROVEMENT

Effectively identifying opportunities for improvement in care transitions involves first identifying the root cause of specific problems. Root causes can be identified through a systematic review of data that indicate an outlier in a particular area. For instance, data may show that patients at a particular hospital have been repeatedly readmitted to the hospital following discharge. Once the problem has been identified, it is necessary to gather additional information to pinpoint the population and implement actions to improve outcomes.

Further data review can help identify the root cause of the problem. For example, it may reveal that the majority of patients being readmitted have hypertension and chronic kidney disease. This allows for a targeted approach to identify whether the patients are being treated by a particular team or specialty at the hospital. In this case, further data review may reveal that all the patients being readmitted have been discharged from the nephrology team at the hospital.

Using this information, the healthcare quality professional can have meaningful conversations with the department to identify ways to prevent avoidable readmissions. This can involve restructuring workflows, providing patient/family education, and/or ensuring that effective and timely follow-up care is established. By addressing the root cause of the problem, it is possible to implement solutions that lead to improved outcomes for patients during care transitions.

HANDOFFS AND TRANSITIONS OF CARE

During handoffs and transitions of care, patients are particularly at risk because critical information may be forgotten or overlooked. The CPHQ should promote the use of a systematic method of communication to be used during handoff procedures to ensure that information is organized and complete. Handoff procedures should be documented and adequate time allowed for communication, including questions from the receiving party. The SBAR (situation-background-assessment-recommendation) tool is commonly used for handoff. The primary purpose is to promote patient safety by ensuring that all pertinent information is conveyed:

- **Situation**: Name, age, overseeing physician, diagnosis.
- **Background**: Brief medical history, co-morbidities, review of lab tests, current therapy, location of IVs, vital signs, pain, special needs, educational needs, and discharge plans.
- **Assessment**: Review of systems; status of lines, tubes, and drains; and completed tasks, needed tasks, and future procedures.
- **Recommendations**: Review plan of care, medications, precautions (restraints, falls), treatments, wound care.

Organizations utilizing SBAR should have guidelines that advise staff exactly what should be covered in each element and a worksheet the providers can utilize to organize information.

HEALTH UTILIZATION AND THE CARE CONTINUUM

A number of different factors must be considered regarding health utilization:

- **Medical necessity**: Care provided to patients should be both necessary and appropriate for the patient's condition and needs.
- **Provision of care**: Treatment and care should be based on evidence-based practice to provide the most efficient, effective, and cost-effective care.
- **Time frame**: Care should be provided in a timely manner and within the timeframe of established benchmarks.
- **Regulatory requirements**: All regulatory requirements must be met in relation to both provision of care and reporting.
- **Drug utilization**: Drug use must be appropriate and outcomes monitored. Medications should be reconciled and polypharmacy avoided when possible. Cost of drugs should be considered as part of the prescribing process.
- **Patient safety issues**: The Joint Commission's National Patient Safety Goals/National Performance Goals should be monitored and the organization's score assessed with the goal of improving safety outcomes and exceeding benchmarks.
- **Patient insurance and resources**: The patient's ability to pay for care and to have necessary support should be considered as part of the plan of care.

COLLABORATING WITH STAKEHOLDERS

Care transitions refer to moving a patient from one setting of care to another. During these transitions, it is crucial for all parties involved to communicate effectively as responsibility shifts. This helps to avoid the risk of adverse events. To support effective care transitions, multidisciplinary collaboration and coordination are critical. For instance, if a patient is transitioning from the hospital to home, it is necessary to involve the hospital physician(s) and nursing staff, the patient's primary care provider, the patient's pharmacy, case and/or care management, and the patient's caregiver(s).

To ensure successful transitions and positive outcomes, several critical considerations should be taken into account. This includes communicating with all parties involved about required follow-up care, symptoms to watch out for that may indicate a problem, medications prescribed to complete/update the medication reconciliation, and points of contact should any concerns arise. Effective communication among all stakeholders is key to ensuring smooth care transitions and preventing any negative outcomes.

Health Data Analytics

Data Management Systems

EVALUATING AND DEVELOPING DATABASES

Databases are computerized file structures that contain organized and accessible stored data. Relational databases, which are built on a multiple table structure with each individual item on a table having a unique identifier, are the most common type. When building a database, one of the first steps to ensuring adequate data is to conduct a requirements analysis, which can involve eliciting information about data through case studies, interviews, focus groups, and observations. Identifying the types of data and the types of interaction with the data is necessary to help determine the data needed because data input must result in desired output. A database may become inflated in size because of redundancy, so eliminating redundancy is essential. The CPHQ can provide input to identify those attributes that are key to identification and those that provide information or provide both identification and information. Then, redundant identification attributes can be removed.

EVALUATING AND DEVELOPING REGISTRIES

Registries are collections of secondary data about specific patient diagnoses, treatment, procedures, and/or conditions. A healthcare organization may develop a number of different registries in order to collect data and to make the data available to researchers as well as to track follow-up care. The CPHQ often has an active role in determining which registries to compile and the case definitions for inclusion in the registry. Common registries include those tracking data on cancer, trauma, congenital defects, diabetes, cardiac conditions, HIV, transplants, and immunizations. Once the registry is established and the case definition completed, the CPHQ may develop protocols for case finding and submission of data. Some registries, such as the cancer registry, are mandated by law, but others are determined by institutional need. Data elements vary according to the type of registry but may include specific demographic information, diagnosis, treatment, stages (when appropriate), status codes, and functional status.

BIG DATA

As the healthcare industry continues to evolve, the ability to access and analyze large sets of information is a critical component for organizations to guide data-driven decision-making. **Big data** is a term used to describe data with large volume, velocity, variety, and veracity. Utilizing this information effectively allows for a better understanding of patient populations and the required care to improve health outcomes.

With the enactment of the **Health Information Technology for Economic and Clinical Health Act (HITECH)** in 2009, federal funds were authorized to expand adoption of the Electronic Health Record (EHR) to improve health care delivery systems. EHRs are patient records stored in a digital format. To receive incentives associated with HITECH's EHR implementation, organizations had to demonstrate compliance with the components of **meaningful use**. Meaningful use, also referred to as the EHR Incentive Program, requires providers to demonstrate integration of the EHR through meeting specific metrics related to improving quality and health outcomes through care coordination and population health, engaging patients in their care, and maintaining privacy.

Big data has become increasingly important as the focus on population health and value-based care continues to grow. Healthcare quality professionals must remain vigilant regarding big data, thoroughly understanding the complexities involved with information sourced from different systems, often in an unstructured format, and develop the skills needed to analyze data and identify actionable next steps.

Performing/Coordinating Data Inventory Listing Activities

To perform or coordinate data inventory listing for information management:

- Assemble a team that includes members knowledgeable about data management and assign them to the inventory.
- Develop a procedure and a reporting grid that includes the type of data, its source, reasons for collection, the receiver, storage method, and its uses.
- Inventory from the top down, because the organization has multiple sources of data.
- Catalog data in this order:
  - **Accreditation** (e.g., core measures)
  - **Licensure** (e.g., infection rates and staffing ratios)
  - **Contracts** (e.g., utilization costs)

Departmental Data Collection

Individual units

When collecting data for individual units, consider the following:

- Include everything that is counted, even if it simply involves a clerk counting the use of Foley catheters to facilitate ordering supplies because this data relates to other measures, such as urinary infection rates.
- Once the inventory is completed, assess the grid for duplications, deficits, and unused data.

Performing/Coordinating Data Definition Activities

Data definition activities are a necessary step in performance improvement. Data definition must be completed as part of the planning process and included in the written plan, using input from quality teams or other sources. Every aspect of data collection requires definition. For example, when measuring infection rates, define what constitutes an infection. Save time by incorporating definitions from the CDC, industry, or accreditation standards. For example, use the Joint Commission's definition of infection, with subtypes of iatrogenic, endemic, epidemic, and healthcare-associated infections.

Outcomes are measured by changes in health status, for example:

- A decrease in mortality
- Changes in behavior or knowledge, such as a diet modification used to control diabetes
- Positive surveys indicating satisfaction with treatment

Outcome definitions are especially important, because outcomes allow progress to be assessed. With any measurement, the outcome must indicate what expected change will occur in response to performance improvement activities.

DATA COLLECTION METHODOLOGY

Correct data collection methodology is comprehensive and encompasses all aspects of performance improvement activities. As the data collection coordinator, the CPHQ ensures that the:

- Data collection staff is selected based on their knowledge and access
- Collection begins with a complete inventory of existing data
- Data collection is systematic
- Unnecessary data collection and duplication of effort is avoided
- Interdisciplinary teams who are knowledgeable about the performance improvement process identify sources of data and guide collection
- Triggers are set
- Most effective data collection method is used
- Data is integrated to help identify patterns or trends (organization-wide and departmental)
- Definitions and collection methods used are based on sound principles of epidemiology ensuring the right type of data is collected
- Frequency and duration of data collection is determined based on actual needs

POPULATION AND SAMPLING

A population is a particular group of individuals, objects, or events. Gather data on either an entire population or a subset of a population within a specified time frame. For example, if all cases of a particular disease, all deaths, or all physicians in a particular discipline are measured, it involves an entire population. Defining the population is critical to data collection and the criteria must be established early in the process.

Sampling measures only a subset of a given population and generalizes the findings to the larger target population. Consider the following factors when sampling:

- The sample must have the characteristics of the target population.
- The design of the collection must specify the size of the sample, the location, and time period. Several factors influence sample size, such as the desired level of confidence, population size, research purpose, and design. It is critical to conduct a power analysis to determine the appropriate sample size.
- The sampling technique must ensure that the sampling represents the target population accurately.
- The design of the collection must ensure that the sampling is not biased.

PROBABILITY SAMPLING

Depending on the goal of data collection, different types of sampling or combinations of sampling may be utilized. Sampling should have a confidence level of 95% (.05 level), meaning that there is a 95% chance that the sample represents the population and results can be replicated. **Probability sampling** occurs when there is an equal chance for any member of a group to be part of the sample, allowing generalization of results to the entire population. Probability sampling is usually more expensive than non-probability sampling. There are six sub-types of probability sampling.

Sub-type	Methodology
Cluster	The target population is divided into clusters or groups, and then a number of these groups are selected at random and all members of the population within the selected groups are sampled.
Multi-stage	This method is similar to cluster. However, all members of the population in selected groups are not sampled. Instead, a sampling of the selected groups is used. Use any method for choosing members of a population, such as simple random sampling.
Simple random	The cases in a given population are chosen randomly, using a standard Table of Random Digits. This is the easiest and most commonly used method of sampling.
Stratified	Two-tier sampling. Divide a group into strata (mutually exclusive groups) with two or more homogeneous characteristics. Sample a specified number from each stratum. Thus, outpatient surgery patients with intravenous solutions are sampled by diagnosis, solution, length of stay, or complications.
Systematic (interval) random	Select the first member of the population randomly; select other members at regular intervals. E.g., the desired sampling is 100:500, so the sampling interval is 5 (1 in 5). Choose a random number between 1 and 5 as the random start. Sample every fifth member to a total of 100 members.
Multi-phase	Two phases are required, but more can be used. Obtain data from an entire specified population. Based on that data, obtain further data from a subgroup within the original population.

NON-PROBABILITY SAMPLING

Non-probability sampling is intentionally biased (not everyone has an equal chance of being included) and results cannot be generalized to an entire population. It utilizes qualitative judgment. Sub-types of non-probability sampling include the following:

Sub-Type	Methodology
Convenience	A type of opportunity sampling when those available are sampled, such as all patients in an STD clinic on a Tuesday.
Quota	Utilizes a stratified population that is divided into subgroups (such as male and female) and then a proportion is sampled, such as 5% of females over 16 with HIV. Sometimes specified numbers are counted, such as 50 males and 50 females.
Purposive	Utilizes members of a particular population, such as all women over 60 with breast implants.
Snowball	A subset of convenience sampling used when identifying subjects is difficult. Current subjects recommend additional subjects that meet criteria for sampling.
Expert	Utilizes subject matter experts to gather information from individuals with expertise in the area of study.

Issues with Data Definition and Collection

Data definitions must be based on a solid understanding of statistical analysis and epidemiological concepts. Ensure that data quality is sufficient by confirming that the data is accurate, accessible, comprehensive, and consistent prior to moving forward with performance improvement activities. Specific issues that must be addressed include the 3 S's, 2 R's, and UV:

3 S's	2 R's	UV
Sensitivity: The data must include all positive cases; accounting for variables decreases the number of false negatives. **Specificity**: The data must include only those cases specific to the needs of the measurement and exclude those that are similar but from a different population, decreasing the number of false positives. **Stratification**: Data is classified according to subsets, taking variables into consideration.	**Recordability**: The tool or indicator must collect and measure the necessary data. **Reliability**: Results should be reproducible. There are 2 measures of reliability: 1. Reliability coefficient measures the consistency of a test. A reliability coefficient of 1 indicates perfect reliability. 2. Interrater reliability measures consistency of results when administered by two independent people.	**Usability**: The tool or indicator should be easy to use and understand. **Validity**: Collection must measure the target adequately, so that the results have predictive value. There are three types of validity: 1. Content (face) validity measures the extent to which an instrument measures what is intended to be measured. 2. Construct validity measures the extent to which inferences can be made from the assessment. 3. Criterion-related validity measures the extent to which an accurate prediction or forecast can be made based on the assessment.

Using Computerized Systems to Analyze Data

The analysis of data by hand is impractical and time-consuming, unless the surveyed population is very small. Most statistical analysis utilizes **computer software programs** to automatically analyze the data in a number of different ways and account for risk factors. Software programs save time by generating numeric data, text reports, and graphs simultaneously. The amount and type of data that must be entered into a program varies, according to the type of software and the necessary data for reports that will be generated. If different programs are used to collect and analyze data, they must be compatible, so that data moves intact from one program to another to generate reports. Data-entry design is important: Fields in which numeric data is entered are calculable and fixed numbers (telephone, birth date, medical record numbers, and Social Security numbers) are entered as text.

Selecting Software for Data Collection

Software selection and evaluation of hardware requires knowledge, time, and financial commitment on the part of the organization. The requirements are as follows:

- **Commitment**: Administration and staff must agree to the financial outlay and to the learning curve as part of the strategic plan.
- **Team selection**: Choose an interdisciplinary team with members who are knowledgeable about data, hardware, and software to evaluate the proposed programs. Educate this team about the performance improvement process. Have them conduct a data inventory first, to determine needs organization-wide and avoid duplication.

- **Identification of system requirements for the organization**: Review the whole organization to determine the current extent of its technology (number, types, and locations of computers) and the ability of the technology to interface. Assess organization-wide goals and needs, barriers to implementing an integrated system, and future needs.
- **Identification of user needs**: Gain staff participation through questionnaires, checklists, surveys, group meetings, brainstorming, and wish lists. Relate needs to the strategic plan. Prioritize them to identify essential needs.
- **Assessment of current systems**: Contact the IT department. Find out if:
    o Staff use current hardware well.
    o Proposed software can interface with current software.
    o Downloads are safe and secure data exchange is possible.
    o Data storage is protected to comply with HIPAA.
    o Current computer capacity is adequate.
    o Proposed software is easy to access, input data, and produce reports.
- **Evaluation of vendors**: Internet search, network, and attend conferences about the kind of software needed. Send a Request for Proposal (RFP) to vendors to facilitate comparison. Get references from vendors as evidence that they effectively implemented the proposed program with similar organizations. Vendors must provide a product history that includes:
    o Frequency of upgrades
    o Compatibility with previous software versions
    o Advice about product maintenance and service upgrades
- **Evaluate and compare different software programs**: Perform a software evaluation in relation to the identified needs of the organization. Decide which specifications must be met. Write an RFP to outline the needs of the organization. Although many vendors will not provide a customized response to an RFP unless the budget is large, the team can use it as a guide and checklist during the evaluation process. When comparing software, ask:
    o Does this program meet our organization's requirements?
    o Is it appropriate for medical needs?
    o Is it compatible with our existing hardware?
    o Is it cost-effective, based on our cost/benefit analysis?
    o Can we visit similar organizations that already use this software, to see it in action?
- **Negotiate a contract**: Always review several vendor contracts prior to completing one. Each contract must include provisions for delivery, installation, training, support, liabilities, prices, payment terms, program modifications, and confidentiality. Seek legal advice.

EVALUATING COMPUTER HARDWARE AND SOFTWARE INTENDED FOR DATA COLLECTION AND ANALYSIS

Performance improvement teams must survey, analyze, and take action quickly if outbreaks or clusters of infection occur. Drawbacks that slow their emergency response time include:

- Manual record keeping and reporting
- Lack of integration among existing computer hardware and software programs (e.g., Laboratories use one program, but nursing units use another that is incompatible.)
- High cost of integrating all computer systems and software

Hire a consultant with expertise in medical hardware and software to advise about the best solution to keep data safe, per HIPAA regulations. Before hiring a software designer to create a custom program to meet specific needs, ensure that it can communicate with existing reporting and other software. If the organization buys generic programs and equipment, budget for expensive upgrades every two years, including the time it takes IT to install and teach users about the upgrades. If selecting web-based programs because patches and upgrades download automatically, ensure the workstations are internet capable, and budget for antivirus software. Always review hardware along with software, to ensure the needs and their uses are compatible.

Centralized hardware systems include:

- Mainframes (a large central computer system with terminals)
- Shared systems (leased computers outside the facility)
- Networks with a server and client computers

Decentralized hardware systems are:

- Unattached to a central computer
- Connected by local area networks (LANs) or wide area networks (WANs)
- Linked through the telephone or internet

Evaluate hardware for:

- Cost
- Operating system types
- Type and amount of memory storage (internal hard disk drives [HDDs], CD, digital video discs, shared off-site, web storage, external hard drives, USB flash drives, cloud storage or solid-state drives [SSDs])
- Flexibility
- Capability
- Current needs

IMPLEMENTING NEW COMPUTER SYSTEMS

Implementing a new computer system for data collection and analysis requires considerable training and a transitional period:

- **Prepare**: Announce the new system organization-wide before installation. Explain how the system benefits the entire organization and relates to the strategic plan. Provide information to staff tailored to fit each area's needs. Give a timeline for transition to the new system.
- **Train**: The type and need for training varies, depending on the individual's responsibility in relation to the computerized system. Make training hands-on, in small groups, and repeat classes at various times, so staff achieves mastery, rather than familiarity. Provide area managers with additional training (expert user level) to assist them in supervising.
- **Supervise**: Once the system is in place, supervise staff to ensure that it is used correctly. Identify problems in use to modify the training curriculum. Stay alert for problems (e.g., staff visiting porn sites, selling patient information to the media, applying for external jobs during work time, or cyberstalking).

COST OF INCOMPATIBLE DATA ENTRY SYSTEMS

If different computerized data entry systems are not integrated, it increases costs for data collectors and Medical Records. For example, if lab reports and nursing notes use incompatible systems, then data collectors duplicate efforts by transcribing them, and Medical Records must print all patients' charts. Hard copy storage wastes space and requires more clerks. Three ways to enter data are:

- **Manual data entry**, the most common method, which means charting directly into the computer or copy typing written information. Make responsibilities for entering data clear, to prevent backlogs. Thoroughly train staff in correct procedures for data entry. Expect errors due to transpositions and entering data on the wrong chart.
- **Scanners**, programmed to read particular forms, such as those with boxes marked in pencil. Optical character recognition (OCR) software scans hard copies into computerized text, so that external reports can be added to the system without retyping.
- **PDAs**, which transfer data collected in the field to a desktop computer, rather than re-entering data from forms by hand.

USING EPIDEMIOLOGICAL THEORY IN DATA COLLECTION AND ANALYSIS

Epidemiology studies the relationship between the frequency and distribution of diseases to determine causes, especially of infectious outbreaks and poisonings. The Society for Healthcare Epidemiology of America (SHEA) is an industry leader in promoting the use of epidemiology for healthcare to reduce infections and improve quality of care. Epidemiology focuses on populations or cohorts of patients, rather than on individuals, so it is especially valuable in relation to data collection and analysis. Use epidemiological data to:

- Assess and compare different clinical practices
- Determine good system design
- Develop criteria for measurement, including outcomes and comparative analysis of data
- Design quality control measures
- Document response to changes

GENERATION, ANALYSIS AND VALIDATION OF EPIDEMIOLOGICAL SURVEILLANCE DATA

Most generation of data is from available resources, such as admissions records, questionnaires, interviews, medical records, public health reports, and laboratory reports. In some cases, data generation is part of the surveillance process. For example, urine cultures may be done routinely as part of a surveillance plan, or threshold rates may generate further testing. Perform **analysis** in a timely manner, because it is especially important for the detection of outbreaks. The type of analysis depends on the expected outcomes and the purpose of surveillance. **Validation** of data is an ongoing process. Review all steps in the generation and analysis of data regularly, especially when threshold rates are exceeded. If, for example, an apparent outbreak of antibiotic-resistant bacteria is detected in wound cultures, then validate the nurses' swab collection procedure and the laboratory technologists' culture plating procedure, to ensure that the outbreak is not a pseudo-epidemic caused by faulty techniques or deviations in Infection Control.

USING RISK STRATIFICATION IN EPIDEMIOLOGICAL SURVEILLANCE STUDIES

Risk stratification involves statistical adjustment to account for confounding issues and differences in risk factors. Confounding issues are those that confuse the data outcomes, such as trying to compare different populations, different ages, or different genders. For example, if there are two physicians and one has primarily high-risk patients and the other has primarily low-risk patients, the same rate of infection (by raw data) would suggest that the infection risks are equal for both physicians' patients. However, high-risk patients are much more prone to infection, so in this case, risk stratification to account for this difference would show that the patients of the physician with low-risk patients had a much higher risk of infection, relatively speaking. Risk stratification is also used to predict outcomes of surgery by accounting for various risk factors (including ASA score, age, and medical conditions). Risk stratification is an important element of data analysis.

TARGETED SURVEILLANCE

Targeted surveillance is limited in scope, focusing on particular types of infections, areas in the facility, or patient populations. It is less expensive than hospital-wide surveillance and may provide more meaningful data, but clusters of infection outside the survey parameters are missed. Targeted areas are picked based on characteristics such as frequency of infection, mortality rates, financial costs, and the ability to use data to prevent infections:

- **Site-directed targets** find particular sites of infection, such as the bloodstream, wounds, or urine.
- **Unit-directed targets** select particular service areas of the hospital, such as intensive care units or neonatal units.
- **Population-directed targets** scrutinize high-risk groups, such as organ transplant patients.
- **Limited periodic targets** combine hospital-wide surveillance of all infections for one month in each quarter, followed by site-directed targets for the rest of the quarter. This increases the chance of detecting clusters of infection, but those that fall outside of the hospital-wide surveillance months are still missed.

DEVELOPING OBJECTIVE PERFORMANCE MEASURES

The development of objective performance measures is critical to monitoring performance improvement. Most organizations have many types of data, but often it is not in a usable form for performance improvement. Identify data needs first. Categories of performance measures include those needed for:

- **Strategic planning** (specific to the organization)
- **Regulations** (to meet state or federal requirements)
- **Contractual agreements** (as in managed care)

Consider all three of these categories when developing performance measures, to avoid duplication, and to ensure that the data collected will evaluate the effectiveness of the organization. The data provided should directly relate to functions and processes. Generally, two types of measurements are required:

- **Outcomes**, which show how the organization is performing and whether or not goals are being achieved. For example, data may measure mortality rates in a Neonatal Intensive Care Unit.
- **Processes**, which show if the organizational systems/functions are working effectively. For example, data may measure compliance with core measures for accreditation.

SELECTING PERFORMANCE MEASURES

Below are areas of concern when selecting performance measures:

- **Responsibility for selection**: Each team should select appropriate performance measures. There may be a number of different teams selecting measures for different levels, such as organization-wide data, as opposed to departmental data. These teams are usually interdisciplinary and members have training or expertise in utilizing performance measures.
- **Clear understanding**: Functions, processes, and variables that may affect outcomes require standardized language, a glossary, and consistent training.
- **Identification of purpose and utilization**: Data may be used to assess quality, for accountability, or for research.
- **Review and inventory**: There must be current, available data within the organization's databases to determine what can be utilized.
- **Measures**: Determine the numerators, denominators, and measures that will be used. Assess the measures for their reliability and validity and document these findings. Post the definitions, and list reasons for their choice and references for each measure.

SELECTING OUTCOME MEASURES

Process and outcomes are equally important in performance improvement. Consider whether to focus on the process or the outcome. Establish both a long- and a short-term focus for outcomes.

- **Short-term outcomes** show results directly related to the process, allowing for modifications of the process.
- **Long-term outcomes** relate more to general quality of care and patient satisfaction, and are used retrospectively to evaluate the process or plan for future care.

Outcomes do not directly assess process, although they serve as an indicator that a process may be effective or ineffective, requiring further study or modification of process. Planners focus on identifying three types of **outcome measures**:

- **Clinical**: Determines if there are positive results from clinical interventions
- **Customer functioning**: Includes indicators of ability to perform
- **Customer satisfaction**: Includes meeting expectations and needs

BALANCED SCORECARD

The balanced scorecard (designed by Kaplan and Norton) is based on the strategic plan, and provides performance measures in relation to the mission and vision statements, and goals and objectives. A balanced scorecard includes not only the traditional financial information, but also includes data about customers, internal processes, and education/learning. Each organization can select measures that help to determine if the organization is on track in meeting its goals. These measures may include:

- **Customers**: Types of customers and customer satisfaction
- **Finances/business operations**: Financial data may include funding and cost-benefit analysis
- **Clinical outcomes**: Complications, infection rates, inpatient and outpatient data, compliance with regulatory standards
- **Education/learning**: In-service training, continuing education, assessment of learning and utilization of new skills, research

- **Community**: Ongoing needs
- **Growth**: Innovative programs

Measures indicated on a balanced scorecard are compared to a target value based on internal or external benchmarks. **Benchmarking** is a strategy that involves comparing performance to others to drive performance improvement initiatives. If the scorecard is adequately balanced, it will reflect both the needs and priorities of the organization itself, and also those of the community and customers it serves.

Dashboard

A digital dashboard, like the dashboard in a car, provides an overview of an organization. A dashboard is an easy to access and easy to read computer program that integrates a variety of performance measures or key indicators into one display, usually with graphs or charts. It might include data regarding patient satisfaction, infection rates, financial status, or any other measurement that is important to assess performance. The dashboard provides a running picture of the status of the department or organization at any point in time, and may be updated as desired—daily, weekly, or monthly. An organization-wide dashboard provides numerous benefits:

- Broad involvement of all departments
- A consistent and easy to understand visual representation of data
- Identification of negative findings or trends so that they can be corrected
- Availability of detailed reports
- Effective measurements that demonstrate the degree of efficiency
- Assistance with making informed decisions

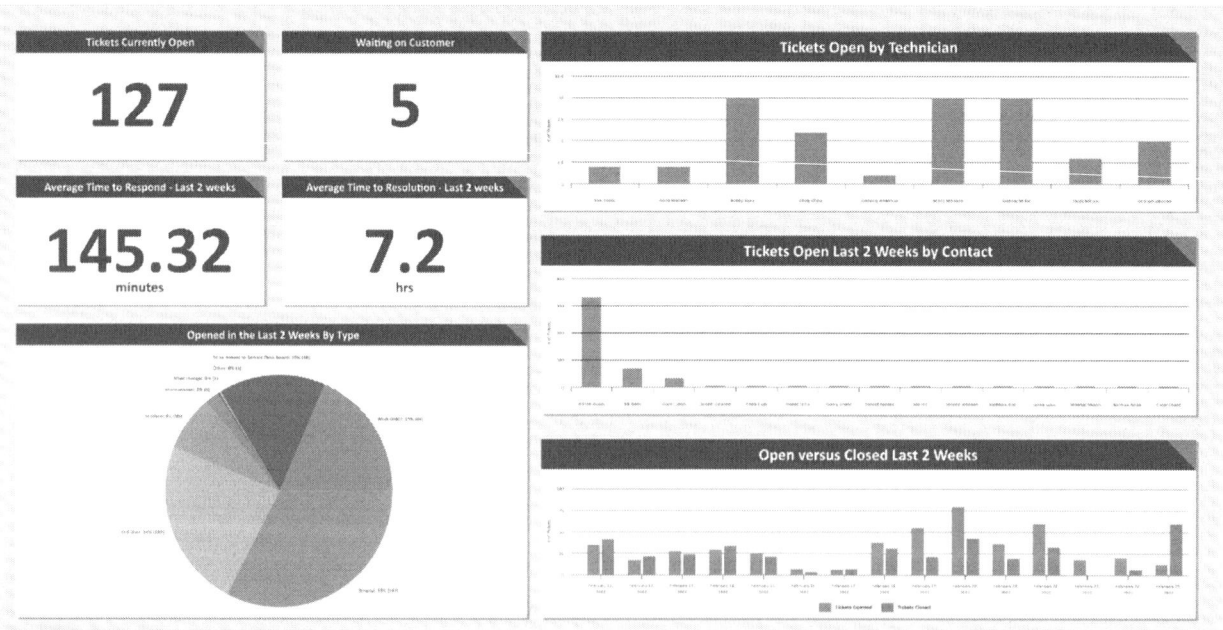

Triggers

Triggers are mechanisms or signals within data that indicate when further analysis or prioritizing must be done, such as case reviews or root-cause analysis. Select triggers for each measure of performance.

Data triggers include:

- **Sentinel events**: Permanent harm or severe temporary harm (for instance, unexpected death or major impairment) occurring because of a process or system deficiency.
- **Adverse events (AE)**: An unintended, unfavorable, iatrogenic occurrence that is life-threatening, or requires inpatient hospitalization, or extends the patient's length of stay, or causes a birth defect or lasting disability.
    - **Preventable adverse events** occur due to failure or error.
    - **Ameliorable adverse events** are not preventable but could have been less severe with proper procedure.
    - **Adverse events due to negligence** occur when care is below standards.
- **Close calls** are patient safety events that do not reach the patient but identify a potential opportunity for improvement.
- **Performance rate**: Pre-established level of performance in a particular measure.
- **Rate change**: A pre-established change over a specified time period.
- **Difference between groups**: A pattern of disparity between specified groups.
- **Specified upper and lower control limits about a mean**: Guardrails establish an acceptable range of variation, usually set by standard deviation methods.

External triggers include:

- Feedback from staff, internal and external customers
- Strategic planning initiatives
- Practice guidelines
- Benchmarks
- Research

IDENTIFYING EXTERNAL AND INTERNAL DATA SOURCES

As part of the data inventory process, all sources of data must be identified, including external and internal data sources. **Internal data sources** are those that originate within the organization. These are numerous and some are easy to overlook, so review all departments for data. **External data sources** originate outside the organization and may reflect activity within or outside the organization.

Internal sources	External sources
Patients' records	Reference databases
Patient and staff surveys	Accreditation reports
Medication records	CDC reports
Clinical review reports (medication use, mortality rates, and autopsy reports)	State or nationally-identified best practice reports
Admissions data (demographics)	Scientific and medical literature reviews
Laboratory reports	State reviews
Observation reports	Threshold data
Infection Control reports	Comparative data
Team and case management reports	Sentinel event alerts
Financial statements	Third-party (payer) reports
Environmental safety reports	National guidelines
Minutes of meetings	
Utilization review reports	

Measurement and Analysis

INTERNAL AND EXTERNAL VALIDITY

Many surveillance plans are most concerned with **internal validity** (adequate, unbiased data properly collected and analyzed within the population studied). However, studies that determine the efficacy of procedures or treatments should also have **external validity** (the results should be generalized and true for similar populations). Replicating the study with different subjects, researchers, and under different circumstances should produce similar results. For example, some people are excluded from a study, so that instead of randomized subjects, the subjects are highly selected. When data is compared with another population in which there is less or more selection, results are different. The selection of subjects, in this case, interferes with external validity. Part of the design of a study should include considerations of whether or not it should have external validity, or whether there is value for the institution based solely on internal validity.

QUALITATIVE AND QUANTITATIVE DATA

Both qualitative and quantitative data are used for analysis, but their focus is quite different:

- **Qualitative data**: Data are described verbally or graphically, and the results are subjective, depending on observers to provide information. Interviews may be used as a tool to gather information, and the researcher's interpretation of data is important. Gathering qualitative data is time-intensive, and it usually cannot be generalized to a larger population. Qualitative information gathering is useful at the beginning of the design process for data collection.
- **Quantitative data**: Data are described in terms of numbers within a statistical format. Quantitative information gathering occurs after the design of data collection is outlined, usually in later stages. Tools may include surveys, questionnaires, or other methods of obtaining numerical data. The researcher's role is objective.

DATA NEEDED FOR ANALYSIS TO ASSIST WITH STRATEGIC PLANNING

Four types of data must be analyzed and summarized to assist with strategic planning:

- **Medical/clinical** information is patient-specific and includes patient history, diagnosis, treatment, laboratory findings, consultations, care plans, physician orders, signed informed consents, and advance directives. The medical record should include records of all procedures, a discharge summary, and emergency care records.
- **Knowledge-based** information includes the following:
    - Methods that ensure staff is trained and supported
    - Research
    - Library services and access to information
    - Good practice guidelines
- **Comparison** data makes internal or external comparisons to benchmarks or best-practice guidelines.
- **Aggregate** data includes pharmacy transactions, required reports, demographic information, financial information, hazard and safety practices, and most things not included in the clinical record.

ORGANIZATIONAL TRANSPARENCY

Organizational transparency is a fairly new concept for the healthcare industry, which has been known for concealment of data. Public pressure to make healthcare organizations more transparent arose in response to unnecessary surgery, inflationary costs, high infection rates, and other negative information in the press. The organization must commit to transparency of pricing and quality, so that both staff and patients have realistic expectations of care. Information that should be available in the reports includes:

- Financial **costs** and **profits.**
- **Performance measures**: Clearly outline the factors that are valued and measured.
- **Outcomes**: List both positive improvements and negative failures to improve to demonstrate quality control is in place.
- **Safety records**: Summarize safety concerns for dissemination, but do not identify those involved without their written permission.
- **Medical records** are open to individual patients and guardians.
- **Leadership qualities** that are parameters for promotion.

WEBSITE CONTENT FOR ENSURING ACCURACY IN PUBLIC REPORTING

When designing a website for public reporting, consider the following questions:

- Who is your audience?
- What type of machine will most viewers use to access your site?
- What type of information do they want?
- Are your code and server secured?
- Are copyright and privacy issues addressed?
- Is access open, or are sections restricted through passwords?
- Who will be the contact for viewer feedback in each section?
- Who updates information for each area or department?
- Is the site primarily informational, educational, or both?
- What format and navigation system are best for the audience?
- How much and what type of direct marketing is included?
- Do interactivity and hi-res graphics slow down page loading?
- Are your typeface and language readable by a large audience?
- What technology is supported (e.g., PDF, Flash, cookies, hit counters, forms, encryption, online credit card payments)?
- Is the site well-designed and easy to use?

ORGANIZING THE AGENDA, REPORTS, AND MINUTES FOR COMMITTEE MEETINGS

Committee meetings provide an opportunity to share data findings with key members of the organization. The agenda, reports, and minutes of a meeting should be recorded accordingly:

- **Agenda**: Distribute the agenda electronically to all interested parties 2–3 days prior to a meeting. Itemize the agenda and include the names of people giving or receiving reports. List approximate times for discussion beside each item, especially if there are many agenda items. If the agenda is for a report to upper management or the governing board, summarize the results of performance improvement activities with a dashboard.
- **Reports**: Schedule reports early in the meeting to allow for discussion, as they may relate to other agenda items. Prepare an electronic slide presentation or use an overhead projector to summarize complex issues.
- **Minutes**: Distribute minutes within 2–3 days after the meeting. Minutes must include brief summaries of each agenda item.

If the organization does not already have standard formats, save time by downloading easy-to-use agendas, reports, slide presentations, and minutes templates from the internet.

AGGREGATION AND SUMMARY OF DATA

Data must be aggregated and summarized for correct analysis of results. Identify those responsible individuals or groups, and the time frame for processing and reporting the data. As the data is collected, display the data on a dashboard or in another manner that demonstrates the type of problems, their extent, and causes. Write a report that summarizes findings and reaches conclusions based on the data. Display data in a graph to make it accessible. Performance improvement professionals must generate reports on a regular basis. Choose monthly, quarterly, or annually, depending on the size of the institution and the population numbers or device days. Statistics must include adequate denominator data for meaningful analysis, which can delay report generation.

CHARTS AND GRAPHS

GRAPHS

Presenting data in the form of charts and graphs provides a visual representation of the data that is easy to comprehend. There are basically 3 types of graphs:

- **Line graphs** have an x- and y-axis, so they are used to show how an independent variable affects a dependent variable. Line graphs show a time series, with time usually on the x (horizontal) axis.

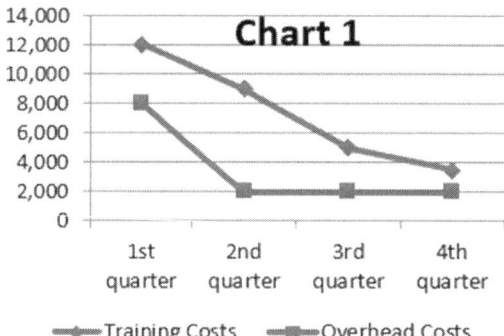

- **Bar graphs** compare and show the relationship between two or more groups. The graphs show quantifiable data as bars that extend horizontally, vertically, or stacked. Bar graphs compare data from different populations or from one time period to another.

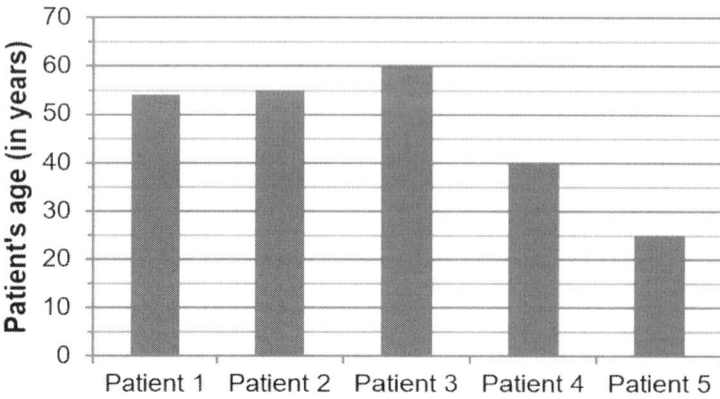

- **Pie charts (circle graphs)** show what percentage an item pertains to the whole. Use a pie chart to show distribution of resources or personnel.

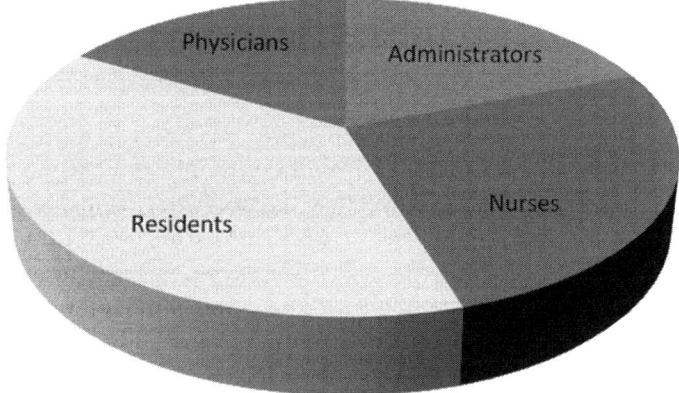

Common chart and graph software programs are Microsoft Excel, Corel Quattro Pro, and Quicken.

Pareto Charts

A Pareto chart is a combination vertical bar graph and line graph. Typically, bar graph values are arranged in descending order. For example, if incidences of bloodstream infections are plotted by unit, then the unit with the largest number appears first on the left. A line graph superimposed over the bar graph shows what accumulated percentage of the total is represented by the elements of the bar graph. Thus, if 50 infections occurred in the ICU, and that represented 30% of the hospital's total infections, the line graph starts at 30%. If 40 infections occurred in the Transplant Unit, the line graph shows 54%. Pareto charts demonstrate the most common causes or sources of problems, and have given rise to the 80/20 rule: 80% of the problem often derives from 20% of causes.

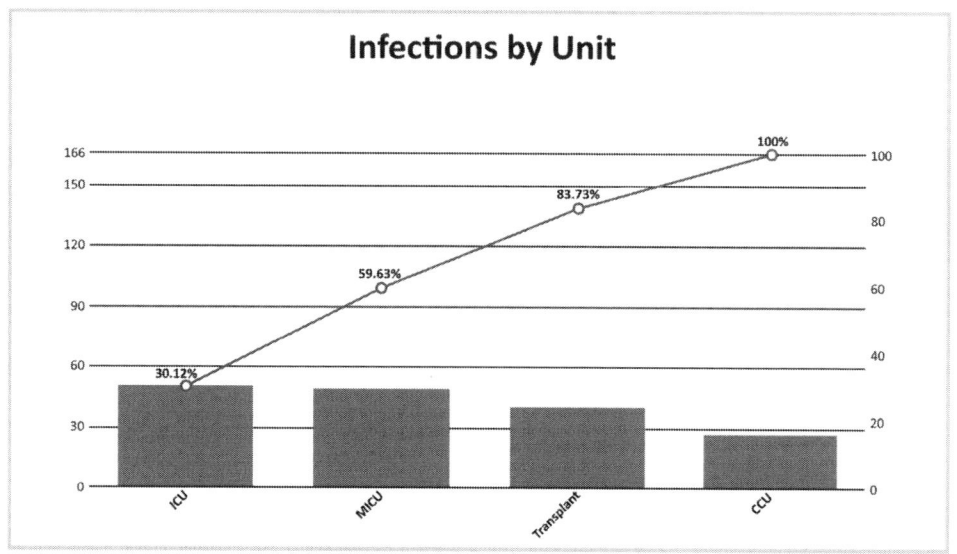

FLOW CHARTS

A flow chart is a quality improvement tool used to provide a pictorial or schematic representation of a process. When searching for solutions to a problem, analyze each step in a process and post it on the flow chart. Use the following standard symbols:

- Parallelogram: Input and output (start/end)
- Arrow: Direction of flow
- Diamond shape: Conditional decision (Yes/No or True/False)
- Circles: Connector joining two parts of a program; divergent paths with multiple arrows enter, but only one arrow exits

Flow goes from top to bottom and left to right. Flow charts help audiences visualize how a process is carried out and examine a process for problems. Flow charts are used to plan a process before its inception. Flow charts demonstrate critical pathways to outline treatment options and paths related to findings. Examples of flow chart programs are Microsoft Visio, Corel Flow, and ABC Flowcharter.

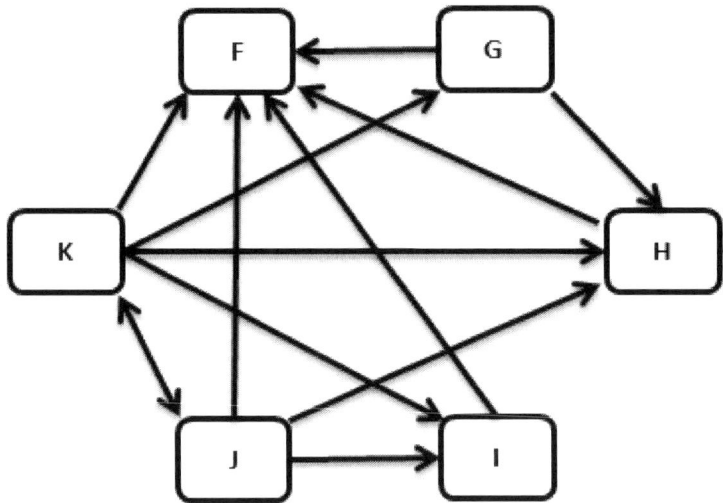

ISHIKAWA FISHBONE DIAGRAM

The Ishikawa fishbone diagram resembles the head and bones of a fish. It is an analysis tool that determines cause and effect and is used for brainstorming. In performance improvement, it identifies root causes. Label the "head" with the problem (effect). Label each "bone" with one of these categories (causes):

- **M** for manufacturing, methods, materials, manpower, machines (equipment), measurement, and Mother Nature (environment)
- **P** for people, prices, promotion, places, policies, procedures, products, and administration
- **S** for service, surroundings, suppliers, systems, and skills

The categories serve only as a guide and are selected and modified as needed.

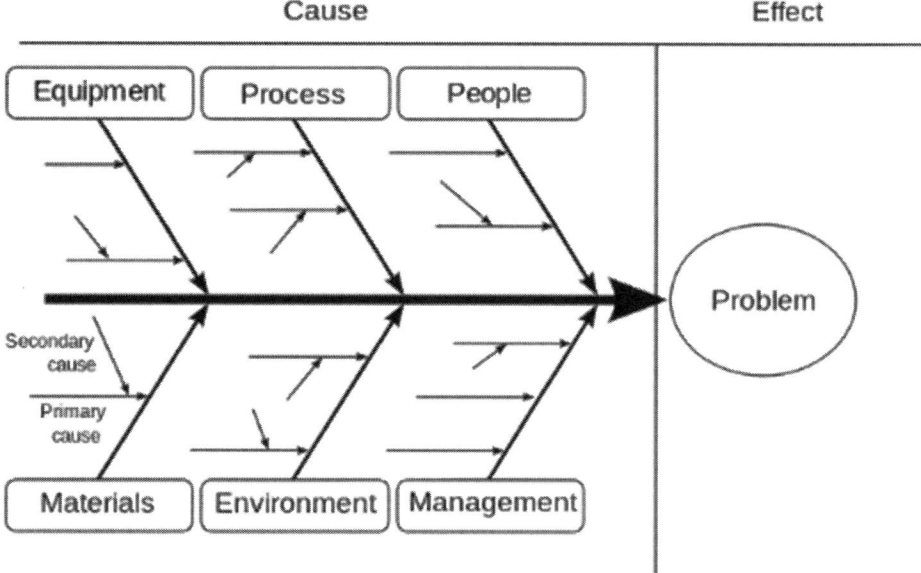

RUN CHARTS

The run chart is a type of line graph with a horizontal x-axis (independent variables) and vertical y-axis (dependent variables, outcomes). The run chart provides a running record of a process over time when a horizontal median line is added. A run is a sequence of data points on one side of the median line, ending when the line crosses the median. Runs should be color coded. For example, a run chart may plot the number of urinary infections by month for a one-year period with increased runs indicated by a different color. Record data for a long enough period, so that normal variations are not misconstrued as significant runs. Note that shifts, trends, patterns, and cycles are defined relative to the total number of data points, so fewer total data points require fewer data points to define each of them.

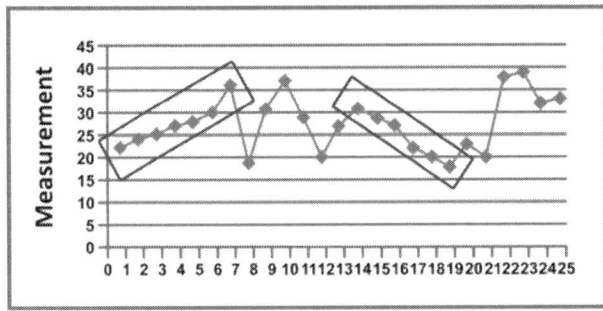

Trends Example

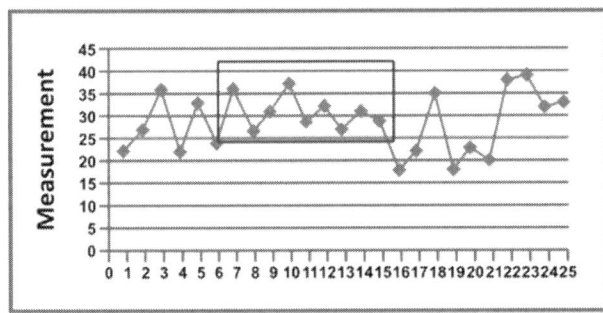

Shifts Example

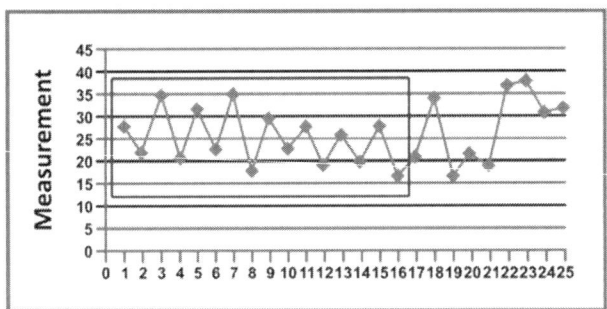

Alternating Example

As an example, run charts with more than 25 data points demonstrate the following:

- **Shifts**: 7 or more consecutive data points all above or all below the median
- **Trends**: At least 5 consecutive data points in either ascending or descending order or at least 6 with more than 20 total data points
- **Patterns**: 8 or more similar fluctuations
- **Cycles**: Up and down variation forming a sawtooth pattern with 14 successive data points, suggestive of a systemic effect on the data. If the trend is related to common cause variation, the variation may be demonstrated with 4–11 successive data points
- **Astronomical value**: A data point unrelated to other points indicates a sentinel event or special cause variation

If any of these changes appear, they point to specific causes that require investigation.

CONTROL CHARTS

The control chart is similar to the run chart but has a mean line (center line) as well as upper and lower control limit lines, based on an expected normal distribution. Every process has some normal variation (common cause or random variation), so the control limits may need to be adjusted over time as more data is collected. Control limits are set at three standard deviations (3σ) above and below the center line and are divided into three equal zones.

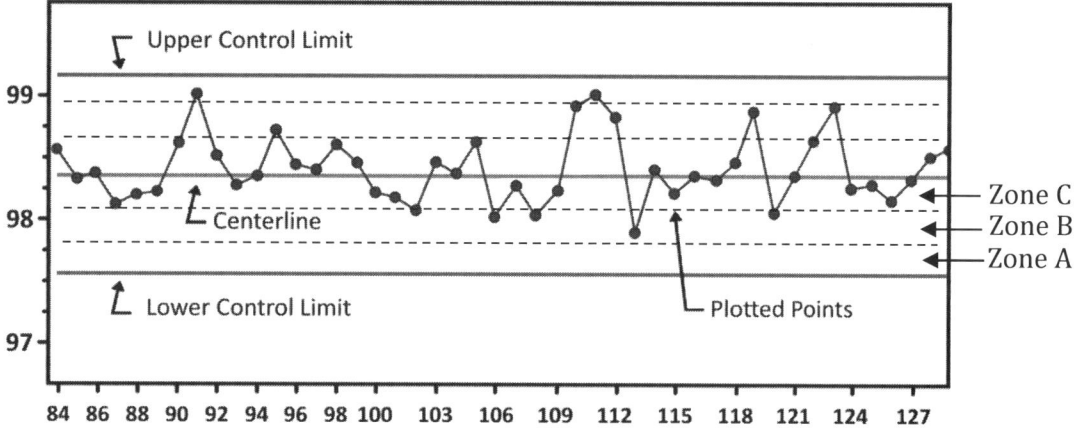

There are several events that should trigger a review to determine if the control limits need to be adjusted or if there is special cause variation taking place that needs to be addressed by modifying the process. The thresholds that trigger these reviews vary by organization. The specific NAHQ recommendations will be noted when applicable. Note that many of these triggers will be ambiguous, in that it will not be clear whether there is special cause variation or the control limits are simply not tuned correctly, so the CPHQ will need to exercise good judgment in determining this and taking the correct actions in response.

EXTREME VALUES

Any data point that falls outside of the 3σ control limits is potentially cause for concern and should be reviewed (**NAHQ standard**).

SHIFTS

Multiple data points that fall more than 2σ from the center line (on the same side) are likely also a cause for concern. NAHQ's standard is that **2 out of 3 consecutive data points that fall outside the 2σ line** is cause for review. Some organizations consider a string of 4 out of 5 consecutive data points more than 1σ from the center line (again, on the same side) to be cause for a review, but NAHQ does not include this trigger.

Another type of shift occurs when several consecutive data points fall above the center line or below the center line. For any given interval, normal random variation would be expected to cause about half of the data points to be on each side of the center line, so if there are an overwhelming number of data points on the same side of the center line, this warrants investigation. NAHQ's standard is that **8 consecutive points on one side of the center line** is cause for review.

TRENDS

Even if the data points have not yet exceeded the control limits, it may be possible to see trends that indicate an extreme value is coming. A run of consecutively increasing or decreasing data points is one such trend. NAHQ's standard is that **6 or more consecutive increasing or decreasing data points** is cause for review.

Patterns

There are several data patterns that do not qualify for any of the previously mentioned triggers that may nonetheless indicate the need for a review. For example, an excessive number of alternating (increasing, then decreasing) data points may indicate that something affecting the process variation is predictable (not random).

Another pattern of interest occurs when an overwhelming number of consecutive data points are very close to (within 1σ of) the center line. While this might seem to be a universally positive occurrence, it is usually an indication that the control limits have been set too wide. If this is the case, they need to be tightened up so that special cause variation can be effectively identified instead of going unnoticed. NAHQ's standard is that **15 or more consecutive data points within 1σ of the center line** is cause for review.

Scattergram

A scattergram graphically displays the correlation between two variables, with one variable represented on the *x*-axis and the other on the *y*-axis.

- Each plotted data point indicates the value of both variables for a given person, event, or time period.
- If the data points show a clear tendency to go up or down when moving left to right across the graph, this indicates correlation (positive or negative).
- **Remember that correlation does not equal causation.** Just because two quantities seem to show a pattern, it does not mean that there is a causal relationship between the two. The correlation could be random, or both quantities could be influenced by some unconsidered third quantity.

Review Video: Data Interpretation of Graphs
Visit mometrix.com/academy and enter code: 200439

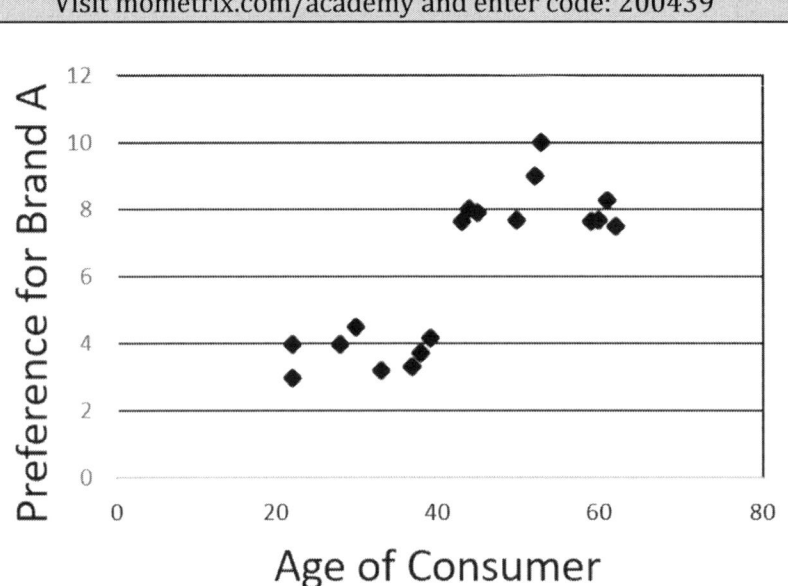

Statistical Testing

When conducting analysis for significance in statistical analysis, there are two types of testing involved: parametric and non-parametric.

Parametric tests, such as regression analysis and t-tests, use continuous data and include assumptions regarding the distribution of the population. **Non-parametric tests**, such as chi-square (X^2), use categorical data and do not make assumptions regarding the distribution of the population.

REGRESSION ANALYSIS

Regression analysis compares the relationship between variables to determine the nature of their correlation, if it exists. There are a few common types of regression analysis that can be performed, but linear regression is the most common. A linear regression determines whether the independent variable (x) can be used to predict the dependent variable (y). For example, a regression analysis would be used to determine if a significant correlation exists between caloric intake and weight. A multiple regression measures the same relationship amongst two or more independent variables (x_1, x_2, etc.) to the dependent variable (y). Regression analysis is essentially the process of comparing a set of real-world data to a mathematical model and assessing how well the data set matches the model.

The strength of a correlation relationship is indicated by the correlation coefficient (r), which ranges from +1 to -1:

- **An r-value of -1** indicates a perfect **negative** correlation: The value of one variable decreases when the value of the other increases.
- **An r-value of +1** indicates a perfect **positive** correlation: Values of both variables increase or decrease together.
- **An r-value close to 0** indicates no correlation: The values of the variables change independently of one another.

The following chart shows a regression analysis of a dataset with a correlation coefficient between 0 and 1:

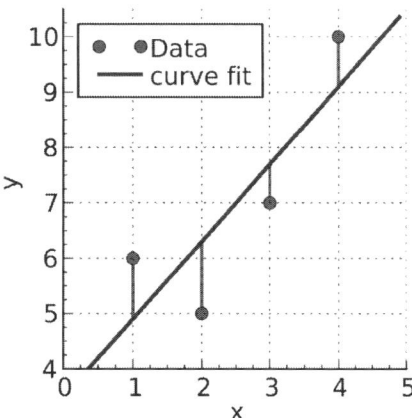

T-TEST

The *t*-test analyzes data to determine if there is a statistically significant difference in the means of both groups. The *t*-test looks at two sets of things that are similar. For example, the *t*-test could compare the average number of miles walked per week by women over 65 who have been diagnosed with breast cancer, as opposed to women over 65 who have not been diagnosed. This example would be considered a **two-sample independent t-test**. If women over 65 who have been diagnosed with breast cancer were tested for cardiovascular fitness, subsequently trained for a marathon, and then tested for cardiovascular fitness post training, this would be a **paired sample t-test**.

CHI-SQUARE TEST

The chi-square (X^2) is a method of comparing rates or ratios. The chi-square test establishes if a variance in categorical data (as opposed to numerical data) is of statistical significance. An example of categorical data is that concerning gender (male vs. female). There are a number of different approaches to chi-square testing, depending upon the type of data, but it is generally used to show if there is a significant difference between groups or conditions being analyzed. For example, use chi-square to compare the rates of surgical infections between two types of surgical procedures.

P VALUES

Surveillance is sometimes confused by randomness. A sudden increase in the infection rate at a facility does not necessarily indicate a systemic problem at the facility, but may simply be a random statistical variation. One useful metric for determining whether an observed effect is the result of random variation rather than a systemic problem is the ***p* value**. The *p* value indicates the likelihood that an observed effect is random, with values ranging from 0 to 1.

- A *p* value **less than 0.05** means that there is less than a 5% probability that the observed effect occurred by chance, meaning that the null hypothesis is rejected. A *p* value **greater than 0.05** means that there is more than a 5% probability that the observed effect occurred by chance, meaning that the null hypothesis is accepted.
- The value **0.05** is generally considered to be the cutoff for **statistical significance**. As a practical matter, policy decisions are typically not made based on studies where the results are not found to be statistically significant.

When reviewing p values to determine significance, there are two types of error that can occur during interpretation:

- **Type 1 error** occurs when the null hypothesis is true, but was rejected.
- **Type 2 error** occurs when the null hypothesis is false, but was not rejected.

It's important to realize though that the *p* value is just one measurement of the significance of probability in a set of data and should be combined with other statistical analyses. A limited outbreak at a small facility may not generate enough data points to attain a statistically significant *p* value, but it can still be epidemiologically important.

INCIDENCE VS. PREVALENCE

Incidence and prevalence surveillance are both hospital-wide surveillance methods. **Incidence surveillance** is ongoing surveillance of infections of all hospitalized patients, recording the number of new infections in a population of patients over a specific period of time. Incidence surveillance is time-consuming and expensive but identifies clusters of infections and allows for risk-factor analysis.

To calculate the incidence rate, use the following formula:

$$\frac{\text{Number of new infections}}{\text{Total population in time period}}$$

Prevalence surveillance involves both period prevalence, which is a specific, pre-determined time period for surveillance, and point prevalence, a specific point in time. Prevalence is the number of nosocomial infection cases active during the period or point of time covered by the survey.

To calculate the prevalence rate, use the following formula:

$$\frac{\text{Number with active infections}}{\text{Total population in time period}}$$

PREVALENCE OF EPIDEMIOLOGICALLY SIGNIFICANT FINDINGS

Prevalence is a good measure of the overall burden of infections/events on a facility, expressing how common they are. Prevalence is often expressed as a percentage.

- In **limited-duration prevalence**, prevalence is looked at retrospectively. It counts all those alive during a period of time (e.g., the past 5 years) who had a particular disease.
- **Complete/lifetime prevalence** counts all those alive at a particular point in time who had the disease at any time in the past or present, whether cured or in current treatment, usually expressed as a ratio of those with the disease, compared to a given population.

RATES, RATIOS, AND RISK RATIOS FOR COMPILING SURVEILLANCE DATA

A **rate** is the number of events per a given population (e.g., 3 infections per 100 patients) or per a time period (e.g., 3 infections per 1,000 device days). These figures are expressed as the **ratios** 3:100 and 3:1,000. Rates and ratios express most infection control data. However, data should be stratified, taking risk factors into account, and different rates derived for different populations for validity.

Risk ratio is the ratio of incidence of infection/disease among those who have been exposed, compared to the incidence among those who have not been exposed. A risk ratio of 1.0 suggests that there is equal risk of infection. A higher number suggests the probability that those exposed will have higher rates. Thus, 1.5 shows that the exposed group is 1.5 times more likely to become infected than those not exposed. A lower number suggests exposure brings less risk of infection (immunity).

CALCULATING PROPORTIONS

A proportion is a subset of ratio that identifies a part of the whole. The event being studied as the numerator data must be a part of the population or database used for the denominator data, for example:

$$\frac{\text{5 urinary infections}}{\text{40 patients with Foley catheters}}$$

Proportions are expressed as either decimals or percentages:

- Calculated as a **decimal proportion**, the above example is $5 \div 40 = 0.125$
- Calculated as a **percentage proportion**, the above example is $5 \div 40 \times 100 = 12.5\%$

Proportion is referred to as a rate when looking at data over a specified period of time. Proportion is frequently used to provide general epidemiological information about specific populations, for example, the number of smokers of different ages in a given population, such as African-American teenage boys.

MEASURES OF AVERAGES

Measures of averages locate the center point of a group of data:

- **Mean** is the average number. However, since distribution can vary widely, the mean may not give an accurate picture. For example, if compiling data and one unit has 20 infections per 100 and the other has 1 infection per 100 (and both have the same total number of patients), the mean (21 ÷ 2) is 10.5 per 100, which has little validity.
- **Median** is the 50th percentile. In order to identify the median of a set of data, the data points must first be arranged in rank/numerical order. For example, consider the following numbers: 3, 9, 7, 15, and 1. First, rearrange the numbers in numerical order: 1, 3, **7**, 9, 15. The number 7 is the median (middle) number. If there is an even number of data points, for instance 14 was added to the data set, then average the two middle numbers, e.g., 1, 3, **7, 9**, 14, and 15. The numbers 7 and 9 are averaged, so the median is 8. If there is an even distribution, the mean and median will be the same. The wider the difference between the two, the more uneven the distribution.
- **Mode** is the number occurring with the highest frequency. There may be bi-modal or tri-modal data sets.

MEASURES OF DISTRIBUTION

Measures of distribution show the spread or dispersion of data:

- **Range** is the distance from the highest to the lowest number. The term interquartile denotes the range between the 25th percentile and the 75th percentile. Report range with median to provide information about both the center point and the dispersion.
- **Variance** measures the distribution spread around an average value. Use variance to calculate the effect of variables. A large variance suggests a wide distribution. A small variance indicates that the random variables are close to the mean.
- **Standard deviation** is the square root of the variance and shows the dispersion of data above and below the mean in equally measured distances. In a normal distribution, 68% of the data is within one deviation (measured distance) of the mean, 95% within 2 deviations and 99.7% within 3 deviations.

RATE COMPARISONS

Comparisons of rates are used to measure or analyze performance. For example, reports of nosocomial (hospital-acquired) infections are often used to compare one facility with another facility or one department in the same facility with another, such as the ICU with the transplant unit. Interpret in-house comparisons carefully, because a higher rate of infection does not always mean patients are at increased risk. To make comparisons meaningful, ensure that data is collected in the same way in different units, and case findings and supporting laboratory tests are consistent and accurate. Risk factors should be similar or results stratified to account for differences in risk factors.

Statistical Significance of Causal Inference (Hill's Criteria)

In epidemiology, a statistical association is not necessarily definitive. Sir A. Bradford Hill (1897-1991) made important contributions to epidemiological research methods by developing criteria to judge a **causal inference**. The more of the following criteria that are met, the more likely that an association is causal (the exposure caused a disease):

- **Strength of association** as measured by a *p* value less than 0.05.
- **Temporality**: Cause must precede event.
- **Consistency of observations**: The same effect occurs in different populations and settings.
- **Plausibility of theory**: The theory is based on sound biological principles.
- **Coherence**: The theory does not conflict with other knowledge/theories.
- **Specificity**: One primary cause for an outcome strengthens causality.
- **Dose relationship**: An increase in exposure should increase the risk.
- **Experimental evidence**: Related experimental research may increase the causal inference.
- **Analogical extension**: That which is true in one situation applies to another

External Benchmarking and Internal Trending

External benchmarking involves analyzing data from outside an institution, such as monitoring national rates of nosocomial (hospital-acquired) infection and comparing them to internal rates. To make this data meaningful, use the same definitions and the same populations for effective risk stratification. Using national data is informative, but each institution is different, so relying on external benchmarking to select indicators for infection control measures or other processes can be misleading. Benchmarking is a compilation of data that may vary considerably if analyzed individually, and its anonymity makes comparisons difficult. Examples of entities used for benchmarking in healthcare include Milliman, CMS, CDC, and large healthcare systems and organizations that assist large healthcare organizations with compiling data.

Internal trending involves comparing internal rates of one area or population with another, such as infection rates in ICU and general surgery. Trending can help to pinpoint areas of concern within an institution, but making comparisons is still problematic because of inherent differences. Use a combination of external and internal data to identify and select reliable indicators.

Opportunities for Decision-Making

Opportunities for decision-making may be evident on analysis of **indicators** (typical cause events, such as infections related to central venous lines) and **outcomes** (rates of infection). Surveillance activities produce both numerator and denominator data. Measure the outcomes against established internal benchmarks or external benchmarks, such as national rates. When it is clear where variances lie, target these particular indicators for improvement. Additionally, observations or other findings may indicate the need for changes in processes. For example, cost-benefit analysis may show that some procedures or processes are not cost-effective, and there are a number of different, cheaper solutions that might achieve the same or better results. Review these alternate solutions, so that the costly processes or procedures become a target for reduction in variable costs to the facility.

Interpreting Specific Types of Data

Interpreting performance productivity reports requires a thorough understanding of statistical processes and measures to make reasoned judgments for using the data. Accurately interpreting data is equally important to collecting it. There are two basic types of data, categorical and continuous.

Categorical Data

Categorical (or **discrete**) data is qualitative and divided into different categories, such as numbers of clinical patients, genders, events, births, and deaths. Categorical data is usually displayed in tables or bar graphs, with the total for each variable referred to as a marginal distribution. Categorical data may be presented as raw numerical data and in ordinal scales (for ranking) or used as numerators and denominators, but the statistics are easier to interpret if they are converted to percentages. Categorical data cannot be fractionated; that is, the data is presented as only whole numbers because, for example, someone cannot be half born. Categorical data can include qualitative information with nominal descriptions rather than numerical data, such as blood types.

Continuous Data

Continuous (**variable**) data is quantitative data measured in both whole and fractional units, such as blood pressure readings, temperatures, and infection rates, and is often used for physical measurements. If data is expressed in fractions or decimals, then it is continuous, not categorical. Categorical data is expressed in whole numbers. Use continuous data to obtain averages (means and medians) and establish ranges and standard deviations for control charts. Continuous data is often used to establish internal benchmarks to compare with external benchmarks, such as national data, to determine how an organization differs, to identify opportunities for process improvement, and to develop effective practice guidelines.

Outcome Data

When interpreting outcome data, keep in mind that there are a number of different types, and some data may overlap:

- **Clinical**: Includes symptoms, diagnoses, staging of disease and indicators of patient health
- **Physiological**: Includes measures of physical abnormalities, loss of function, and activities of daily living
- **Psychosocial**: Includes feelings, perceptions, beliefs, functional impairment, and role performance
- **Integrative**: Includes measures of mortality, longevity, and cost-effectiveness
- **Perception**: Includes customer perceptions, evaluations, and satisfaction
- **Organization-wide clinical**: Includes readmissions, adverse reactions, and deaths

When considering outcome data, focus on the purpose of reviewing the data, rather than on a process or the outcome data itself. The team must analyze the data to understand how process and outcome data interrelate.

Interpreting Performance Productivity Reports

Performance productivity reports provide a wealth of information about the processes within an organization, but interpreting the data requires a thorough understanding of the organization and existing processes. The data may be useful for a variety of purposes:

- **To evaluate clinical processes**: Changes often require cooperation of medical staff, including physician compliance with best practices and core measures, and providing supporting data can be a powerful motivator.
- **To coordinate needs and services across the organization**: Data may, in some cases, be generalized to apply to multiple processes.
- **To assure an acceptable balance of cost-effectiveness and good practices.**

- **To promote a culture of accountability**: Data provides objective information about cause/effect and outcomes.
- **To improve the flow of information**: Data can be used effectively to communicate needs and promote interchange of ideas.

PROCESS VARIATION

When interpreting performance productivity reports, the CPHQ must have a clear understanding of **process variation** to determine whether variations found in the data are within an acceptable range or are cause for concern. Some random variations are normal with patient care processes and patient responses. For example, patients respond differently to the same treatment. Common-cause problems are difficult to resolve and require changes in general processes, but variations can be reduced to a stable level. Assignable causes are identifiable, such as sentinel events, which are traced through root cause analysis. Deal with assignable causes individually, with case-specific reviews to identify and eliminate the cause of the variation. Variations can be positive, and then further study is needed to determine how best to replicate the beneficial practice.

INTEGRATING PERFORMANCE PRODUCTIVITY REPORTS INTO THE PERFORMANCE IMPROVEMENT PROCESS

Performance productivity reports are a beginning point in efforts to improve performance. The reports must be analyzed to determine what areas of improvement have the most impact on strategic goals and outcomes related to goals. Prioritize needs. Use the reports as a basis for improved performance in the following ways:

- **Education and training**: Inform staff about the results of the reports, because making people aware of how well they are doing and what areas need improvement provides an impetus for change. Develop specific training aimed at improving performance according to needs indicated by the reports.
- **Mentoring**: Identify and train staff with strong skills to mentor and assist others in improving performance.
- **Resources**: Productivity reports often highlight resource needs. Supply staff with the equipment and support they need to achieve performance improvement.

NECESSARY INTEGRATION OF THE RESULTS OF DATA ANALYSIS

Integrating the results of data analysis into performance improvement is necessary because attempting performance improvement without data is essentially operating blind. Data should be used not only as the basis for long term strategic planning, but for identifying opportunities for **performance improvement activities** on an ongoing basis. Integration of information includes:

- Identifying issues for tracking.
- Reviewing patterns and trends to determine how they impact care.
- Establishing action plans and desired outcomes based on the need for improvement.
- Providing information to process improvement teams to facilitate change.
- Evaluating systems and processes for follow-up.
- Monitoring specific cases, criteria, critical pathways, and outcomes.

Integrated information assists with case management and decision-making about patient care, as well as improves critical pathways related to clinical performance, staff performance evaluations, credentialing, and privileging.

BENEFITS OF INTEGRATING THE RESULTS OF DATA ANALYSIS

The benefits derived from integrating the results of data analysis into the improvement process are:

- Coordination of management/leadership functions provides more efficient planning.
- Evidence-based care decisions increase cost-effectiveness and improve outcomes.
- Duplication of effort is reduced through the sharing of information, increasing the overall efficiency of the organization.
- Staff utilization is more effective.
- Improved accountability allows for better performance assessment.
- Communication among departments/areas within an organization is improved.
- The use of a common database facilitates tracking of patterns and trends.
- Responses can be tailored to the needs of staff, patients, and the organization as a whole.
- Organizational obstacles are dealt with more efficiently because of supporting data.

INITIAL VS. INTENSIVE ANALYSES

An initial analysis must be conducted for every monitored process. This means identifying team members responsible for the aggregation and analysis of data, specifying timelines for aggregation and analysis of data based on the volumes of customers, services, procedures, and the impact on those involved. Once the timeline is established, the analysis should begin. Data is reviewed for accuracy and reliability and compared both internally and externally to look for trends or patterns. Data is reviewed for evidence of sentinel or individual events for further study. Triggers are set for patient safety or other areas of concern. Trigger events spark an **intensive analysis**, which is used to identify opportunities for improvement, and to identify significant deficiencies and the scope of problems.

Intensive analysis focuses on:

- Sentinel events
- Performance levels outside of normal variations
- Performance levels outside of benchmarks or best practices
- Hazardous conditions
- Medical discrepancies and errors

RELATION OF SELECTION BIAS AND INFORMATION BIAS TO STATISTICAL SIGNIFICANCE

Selection bias occurs when the method of selecting subjects results in cohorts who are not representative of the target population because of an inherent error in design. For example, if all patients who develop urinary infections with urinary catheters are evaluated per urine culture & sensitivities for microbial resistance, but only those patients with clinically-evident infections are included, a number of patients with sub-clinical infections are missed, skewing the results. Selection bias is only a concern when participants in studies are specifically chosen. Many surveillance studies do not involve subject selection.

Information bias occurs when there are errors in classification, so an estimate of association is incorrect.

- **Non-differential misclassification** occurs when there is similar misclassification of disease or exposure among both those who are diseased/exposed and those who are not.
- **Differential misclassification** occurs when there is a differing misclassification of disease or exposure among both those who are diseased/exposed and those who are not.

Identifying Variances That Require Action

To identify variances that require action, first ensure that baseline data is representative of the target population. This requires an initial period of surveillance and review, ideally for one month. Establish threshold rates. Once the baseline is established, analyze new data to identify variances (changes, like an infection increase that indicates an epidemic or a mortality decrease that indicates improvement). Predetermine a trigger for an alert. For example, if infection rates increase 2 standard deviations above the monthly mean, this variance triggers an alert. Alerts may be tied to time, so that an increase over a 3-month period triggers an alert. Once data triggers a variance alert, a statistical analysis must be completed as soon as possible to determine the:

- Relevance of the variance.
- Probability of the variance occurring by chance.
- Statistical significance or insignificance of the variance.

Interpretation of Incident Reports

Incident reports, also called occurrence reports, provide valuable evidence of a problem with process performance. About 50% of incident reports relate directly to medical error. Use incident reports to investigate the incident, provide a guide to change, provide data about occurrences, and provide legal defense related to liability claims. There are four primary types of events related to medical error:

- Near error
- Unsafe activity
- Sentinel
- Adverse

The organization must have a systematic method in place for interpreting incident reports, which involves not only collecting data relating to the reports, but also analyzing the data and utilizing it for educational purposes and performance improvement activities. An important function of interpretation is to determine if the incident could have been prevented, and, if so, what part of the current process failed and what can be done to prevent similar incidents in the future.

Interpretation of Outcome Data

Outcome data guides performance improvement activities because it gives evidence of how well a process succeeds, but not necessarily the reasons; therefore, the CPHQ must evaluate the outcome data to find reasons. Consider these two inherent problems with outcome data when using outcomes for process improvement:

- It is almost impossible to provide sufficient risk stratification to provide complete validity to outcome data
- It is also difficult to accurately attribute the outcome data to any one step in a process without further study

For example: Outcome data shows a decline in deaths in the emergency department, which recently changed its trauma procedures. The outcome data does not take into account the local police station's gang task force, which successfully decreased drive-by shootings and killings by 70% in the catchment area. The CPHQ might assume that changes in the emergency department's trauma procedures altered the outcome data when, in fact, if the data were adjusted for these external factors, the death rate may have increased.

Tie process improvement activities and **outcome data** to each other and assess processes for their cost-effectiveness. For example: An initial cost-benefit analysis determined an intervention was necessary in infection control. The governing board agreed to implement a proposed intervention by investing $93,000 per year, expecting a savings of 5 infections at $27,000 each for a total of $135,000. This comes out to a net savings of $42,000 (135,000 – 93,000). After one year, the CPHQ carefully assesses the outcomes to determine if the intervention met the goal set for it and whether it was cost-effective. They discover that the savings amounted to only 2 infections for a total of $54,000. Thus, the intervention resulted in a net cost to the hospital of $39,000 (93,000 – $54,000).

However, changes in practice should not be based solely on monetary figures. Further analysis must be performed to determine if other variables affected the outcomes. If the hospital opened a transplant unit with additional surgical patients, then the reduction in 2 infections might be impressive. If there is a *Staphylococcus* carrier among the staff, then this might account for additional infections. In some cases, a change of practice is required regardless of the monetary implications.

MODELS OF INTEGRATION

Integrating the results of data analysis into the performance improvement process varies from one type or size of organization to another, depending on the model of integration that the organization uses:

- **Organizational**: Processes for improvement are identified and teams are selected to participate in different areas or departments. Teams report to the same individual, who monitors progress.
- **Functional/Coordinated**: Staff specialties, such as risk management and quality management, are not integrated. They remain separate, but draw from the same data resources to determine issues related to quality of care and efficiency.
- **Functional/Integrated**: Staff specialties remain, but there is cross-training among specialties, and a case management approach to patient care is used, so that one person follows the progress of a patient through the system and coordinates with the various specialties, such as infection control and quality management.

REPORTING INACCURATE DATA

The organization of reporting can result in inaccurate data if:

- **Insufficient information** results from incomplete medical records or lab reports at the time of survey. There may be a failure in the reporting procedure, so that some data is not reported.
- **Evaluation errors** occur when data is available but is overlooked, or its significance is not understood, so that the data is not included in a survey.
- **Insufficient laboratory testing** occurs because the attending physician receives a report that indicates clinically evident infection, but does not follow up to verify it, and threshold rates have not been established to automatically trigger a follow-up.
- **Negligence** makes staff reluctant to verify and report infections and negative events in order to keep their rates artificially low.

Because of differences in the efficiency of collecting data, the facility with the lowest infection rate may be the one with the least accurate collection of data.

Patient Safety

Patient Rights and Patient Advocacy

PATIENTS' RIGHTS

Patients' rights are outlined in standards from the Joint Commission and National Committee for Quality Assurance. Rights include:

- Respect for personal dignity and psychosocial, spiritual, and cultural considerations
- Responsiveness to needs related to access and pain control
- Ability to make decisions about care without coercion, including informed consent, advance directives, and end-of-life care
- Procedures for registering complaints or grievances
- Protection of confidentiality and privacy
- Freedom from abuse or neglect
- Protection during research and information related to ethical issues of research
- Appraisal of outcomes, including unexpected outcomes
- Accessible information about organization, services, and practitioners
- Appeal procedures for decisions regarding benefits and quality of care
- Organizational codes of ethical behavior
- Procedures for donating and procuring organs and tissue for transplants

LIVING WILLS, DNR, AND DURABLE POWER OF ATTORNEY

In accordance with federal and state laws, patients have the right to **self-determination** in healthcare, including decisions about end-of-life care through **advance directives**, such as living wills and the right to assign a surrogate person to make decisions through a **durable power of attorney.** Patients should routinely be questioned about an advance directive when they present at a healthcare organization. Patients who indicate they desire a "do not resuscitate" (DNR) order should not receive resuscitation or heroic measures for terminal illness or conditions in which meaningful recovery cannot occur. Patients and families of those with terminal illnesses should be questioned as to whether the patients are hospice patients. For those with DNR requests, or those who request no heroic measures and withdrawal of life support, staff should provide the patient with palliative, rather than curative measures. Palliative measures include pain control, oxygen supplements, physical comforts and emotional support to the patient and family. Treat religious traditions and beliefs about death with respect.

PATIENT ADVOCACY AND MORAL AGENCY

Use both internal and external resources for patient advocacy and moral agency:

- **Advocacy** is working for the best interests of the patient when an ethical issue arises, despite conflicts with personal values.
- **Agency** is openness and recognition of issues and a willingness to act.
- **Moral agency** is the ability to recognize and take action to influence the outcome of a conflict or decision.

Ethical issues are difficult to assess because of personal bias, so share concerns with internal resources and reach a consensus. Issues of concern include options for care, refusal of care, privacy rights, adequate relief of suffering, and the right to self-determination. Internal resources include the ethics committee and risk managers, who can provide guidance related to personal and institutional liability. External agencies include government agencies, such as the Public Health Department.

> **Review Video: Patient Advocacy**
> Visit mometrix.com/academy and enter code: 202160

RESOLVING ETHICAL AND CLINICAL CONFLICTS

Ethical and clinical conflicts among patients and their families and healthcare professionals are not uncommon. Issues frequently relate to medications and treatment, religion, concepts of truth-telling, lack of respect for the patient's autonomy, limitations of managed care, or incompetent care. Healthcare providers are in a position to easily manipulate patients and their families by providing incomplete information and influencing decisions. The CPHQ questions and listens, acknowledges each person's perspective, and shares different viewpoints. Open communication is critical to resolving conflicts. Ask what steps could be taken to resolve the conflict or how it could be handled differently. This often leads to compromise because it allows for an exchange of ideas and validates legitimate concerns. Sharing cultural perspectives can lead to better understanding. Advocacy for the patient and family must remain at the center of the CPHQ's conflict resolution technique.

PROMOTING AN ENVIRONMENT CONDUCIVE TO ETHICAL DECISION-MAKING AND PATIENT ADVOCACY

An environment suitable for ethical decision-making and patient advocacy does not appear spontaneously during a crisis; it requires planning and preparation. The institution must clearly communicate that nurses are legally and morally responsible for assuring competent care and respecting the rights of patients. Decisions regarding ethical issues often must be made quickly, with no time for contemplation; therefore, immediately discuss ethical issues as they arise. The CPHQ must:

- Ensure the policies and procedures manual clearly defines how to deal with conflicts
- Assemble an active ethics committee
- Provide in-service training
- Discuss ethics at staff meetings

Patients and families need to be part of the ethical environment, and that means empowering them by providing information (print, video, audio) that outlines patients' rights, the procedures for expressing their wishes, and dealing with ethical conflicts. Respect for privacy and confidentiality, and a non-punitive atmosphere are essential.

Incorporating Patient and Family Rights into Action Plans

Patient and family rights must be incorporated into action plans. Design the action plan collaboratively and encourage participation from patients and family members. Include patients and families on advisory committees. Use assessment tools, such as patient and family surveys, to gain insight into the issues that are important to them. Infants and small children cannot speak for themselves, so the CPHQ must act as their advocate. Include not only the immediate family, but also other groups or communities who have an interest in patient care (e.g., local AIDS committee). Many hospital stays are now short-term, so programs must include follow-up interviews and assessments to determine if the needs of the patient and family were addressed in the care plan.

Role Modeling, Teaching, Coaching, and Mentoring

Various approaches can be used to help develop nurses' advocacy, moral agency, and caring practices:

- **Role modeling** takes place when one nurse serves as an ideal example for others, demonstrating the behavior and responses that advocate for the patient and show caring practices. The nurse observes, interviews, attempts to understand the patient/family's perspective, and intervenes to assure that their needs are met.
- **Coaching** is providing staff with tools, responses, or procedures that help them to advocate.
- **Mentoring** is providing professional guidance to a staff member who has questions or concerns, and acting as a resource.

Empowering Patients and Families to Act as Their Own Advocates

Empower patients and families to act as their own advocates by giving them a clear understanding of their rights and responsibilities in print or an audio/video presentation on admission, or as soon as possible thereafter:

- **Rights** include competent, non-discriminatory medical care, respect for privacy, participation in decisions about care, and the right to refuse care. Give clear, understandable explanations of treatments, options, and conditions, including outcomes. Explain transfers, changes in care plans, and advance directives. Give access to medical records, and information about charges.
- **Responsibilities** include providing honest, thorough information about health issues and medical history. Encourage them to ask for clarification if they don't understand the information provided to them and to follow the plan of care that is outlined, or explain why that is not possible. They should treat staff and other patients with respect.

INTEGRATING CONCERNS AND VALUE SYSTEMS INTO A PATIENT'S PLAN OF CARE

The CPHQ must understand what is most important to the patient, family, staff, administrators, and payers in the plan of care. Participants have widely divergent concerns. Integrating their various perspectives is an ongoing effort, as it is impractical to call a participant meeting to discuss each care plan. Identify general concerns and values for the institution or the unit, and individualize them for each patient. For example:

- The child wants her parents to be with her at all times.
- Parents want religious and cultural concerns about medical care to be respected.
- The insurance company wants appropriate, cost-effective treatments.
- Nurses want treatments clearly outlined and carried out competently.
- Nutritionists want the child to have appropriate TPN.
- Radiologists want to minimize the child's exposure to x-rays when placing nasogastric tubes.

An adequate care plan allows all of these concerns to be addressed.

ETHICS AND PAIN MANAGEMENT

Promoting a caring and supportive environment means ensuring that the patient is comfortable. According to Joint Commission guidelines and federal law, all patients have the right to **pain management**, and this applies to infants and children too.

- Assess pain management procedures already in place to determine their effectiveness or need for change
- Establish the minimum standard that should be legally followed
- Ensure a pharmacist, anesthetist, and nurses collaborate on an updated pain management policy and procedure
- Clarify responsibility for pain control and imbed this in the standards of practice, e.g., involve oncologists, surgeons, rheumatologists, and other specialists who prescribe analgesics and anesthetics
- Train staff about guardrails to reduce pain safely
- Educate patients to understand they are entitled to pain control, rapid response, and the benefits of pain management
- Promote the new pain management policy and procedure organization-wide

Technology Solutions to Enhance Patient Safety

INFORMATION SYSTEMS

Information systems are used to support daily operations and the decision-making process throughout healthcare delivery systems. They are an efficient way to compile data and ensure that it is easily accessible when needed to move forward with decisions impacting patient safety, quality, or cost within an organization. Two information systems critical to healthcare operations include the following:

- **Administrative (non-clinical) support information systems** consist of financial, human resource, and office components that support daily operations. For example, the financial component would contain payroll, patient accounting, and budgeting, while the human resource component would contain information related to employee records, performance management, and labor analysis.
- **Clinical information systems** are those that support the direct care process. It is important that clinical information systems integrate with administrative information systems to support the best outcome.

CLINICAL DECISION SUPPORT SYSTEMS

Clinical decision support systems (CDSSs) are interactive software applications that provide information to physicians or other healthcare providers to help with healthcare decisions. The programs contain a base of medical knowledge to which patient data can be entered, and an evidence-based inference system provides patient-specific advice. For example, a CDSS may be used in the emergency department so that staff can enter symptoms into the program and, based on the information entered, the CDSS program provides possible diagnoses and treatment options. The CDSS may be used for a variety of purposes:

- Record keeping and documentation, such as authorizations
- Monitoring of patients' treatments, research protocols, orders, and referrals
- Ensuring cost-effectiveness by monitoring orders to prevent duplication or tests that are not indicated by the condition, signs, or symptoms
- Providing support for physician diagnosis and ensuring treatments are based on best practices

The CDSS also integrates financial information to allow for in-depth analysis to further predict performance and assist with critical business decisions to ensure they align with an organization's long-term strategy. For example, when a hospital would like to determine the feasibility of adding a new service line, the CDSS assists with providing meaningful data to support the decision.

COMPUTERIZED PHYSICIAN/PROVIDER ORDER ENTRY SYSTEM

Computerized physician/provider order entry (CPOE) systems are clinical software applications that automate medication/treatment ordering, requiring that orders be typed in a standard format to avoid mistakes in ordering or interpreting orders. CPOE is promoted by Leapfrog as a means to reduce medication errors. About 50% of medication errors occur during ordering, so reducing this number can have a large impact on patient safety. Most CPOE systems contain a clinical decision support system (CDSS) too, so that the system can provide an immediate alert related to patient allergies, drug interactions, duplicate orders, or incorrect dosing at the time of data entry. Some systems can also provide suggestions for alternative medications, treatments, and diagnostic procedures. The CPOE system may be integrated into the information system of the organization for easier tracking of information and data collection. A CPOE system is cost-effective, replaces handwritten orders, and allows easy access to patient records.

BARCODE MEDICATION ADMINISTRATION

Barcode medication administration (BCMA) uses wireless mobile units at the point-of-care to scan the barcode on each unit of medication or blood component before it is dispensed. Scanning ensures the correct medication and dosage are given to the correct patient, eliminating most point-of-administration medication errors. The BCMA system can also be used for lab specimen collection, sorting, and testing. BCMA requires monitoring and input from Pharmacy, as each new barcode must be entered into the system. Additionally, some medications are received in bulk, so when they are dispensed in unit doses, barcodes must be individually attached. Staff must be trained to ensure that BCMA is utilized properly and consistently. The FDA requires drug suppliers to provide barcodes on the labels of medications and biological products (e.g., vaccines). BCMA increases safety for patients by integrating with the medication administration record and the information system of the organization, providing data for assessing performance and performance improvement measures.

RADIO FREQUENCY IDENTIFICATION

Radio frequency identification (RFID) is an automatic tracking system that employs embedded digital memory chips, with unique codes, to follow patients, medical devices, medications, and staff. A chip can carry multiple types of data, such as expiration dates, patients' allergies, and blood types. A chip may be embedded in the identification bracelet of the patient, and all medications for the patient may be tagged with the same chip. Chips have the ability to both read and write data, so they are more flexible than bar coding. The data on the chips can be read by sensors from a distance or through materials, such as clothes, although tags don't apply or read well on metal or in fluids. There are two types of RFID:

- **Active**: Continuous signals are transmitted between the chips and sensors.
- **Passive**: Signals are transmitted when in close proximity to a sensor.

Thus, a passive system may be adequate for administration of medications, but an active system would be needed to track movements of staff, equipment, or patients.

Computerized Notification Systems

The computerized notification system alerts physicians to abnormal laboratory or imaging results. Although this system ensures that alerts are communicated, some results are still lost, and physician follow-up is not always completed, especially in Ambulatory Care, where the physician may not see the patient on a regular basis. These steps improve safety and follow-up:

- Train physicians to check for computerized notices daily. Give clear explanations of the goals, needs, and responsibility for patient safety.
- Set the system to send an automatic notification to the sender when the receiver opens the alert message.
- Set the system to send an automatic second notification to the receiver if the alert message is not opened within a preset period of time.
- Set the system to send an automatic notification to the sender to contact the physician by other means if the second notification is not opened within a preset period of time.
- Monitor and evaluate physicians for compliance.

Electronic Medical Records

The electronic medical record (EMR) is a digital, computerized patient record, often integrated with CPOE and CDSS to improve patient care and reduce medical error. Software applications vary considerably and standardization has not yet been implemented, so the organization must carefully review its current and future anticipated needs against the compatibility of applications to interface with each other to provide for adequate measurements, data collection, reports, retrieval of data, analysis, and confidentiality. Physicians in private practice, especially those in large groups, often employ EMRs, which may be different systems than those used in hospitals. Systems can be customized to meet the needs of the organization, but cost and lack of standardization remain barriers for implementation. However, there is a positive correlation between comprehensive EMR systems and patient outcomes. Quantifiable data about cost-effectiveness is difficult to calculate because savings are often in terms of saved time, fewer interventions, and reduced errors.

Enhancing the Culture of Patient Safety

DEVELOPING AN ORGANIZATION'S CULTURE OF SAFETY

Developing an organization's patient safety culture reduces errors related to medications, treatment, patient care, and other adverse events. Assessment includes reviewing mortality rates, outcomes, best practices, critical pathways, accreditation reports, internal and external benchmarking, and comparative data. To develop a culture of patient safety, the CPHQ must:

- Identify the baseline.
- Establish an ongoing organizational vision directed at patient safety, with commitment by the governing board and upper management to the allocation of financial, personnel, and time resources.
- Establish strategic plans to promote safety.
- Communicate organization-wide about the importance of safety, including education and training.
- Empower staff to identify errors and intervene to reduce risks.
- Identify systemic processes that provide opportunities for improving patient safety.

There are five types of safety cultures:

- **Informed culture** is one where everyone is clear on what is right and wrong.
- **Reporting culture** is one where incidents can be reported without retaliation.
- **Learning culture** is one where an organization encourages growth through learning from mistakes.
- **Flexible culture** is one where an organization is open to change and can quickly adjust as needed.
- **Just culture** is one of shared accountability where unintentional errors are not punished, but rather used as opportunities to learn for the organization.

UTILIZING AHRQ SURVEYS

Begin assessment of the organization's patient safety culture with a survey. The **Agency for Healthcare Research and Quality** (AHRQ) sponsors surveys on patient safety culture (SOPS) for assessing patient safety in different healthcare organizations, including hospitals, nursing homes, and outpatient facilities.

AHRQ's SOPS are suitable for all levels of staff within the organization and are specific to the various health care settings (hospital, medical office, nursing home, community pharmacy, and ambulatory surgery center). The surveys ask questions related to safety, errors in medications and treatments, and incident reporting. They typically take less than 15 minutes to complete, so these surveys could be completed as part of staff meetings or during clinical hours. The surveys use a scale of 1–5, checklists, and narrative responses.

Sections for the hospital setting SOPS include:

- Work area/unit
- Supervisor/manager
- Communication
- Reporting patient safety events
- Patient safety rating
- Hospital/Facility
- Background information
- Comments

EFFECT OF EXTERNAL FORCES ON THE CULTURE OF SAFETY

The patient safety culture constantly evolves in response to new information, technology, and both internal and external forces. The **important external forces** that impact the development of an organization's patient safety culture include the following:

- **External regulations, legislation, and healthcare initiatives**, such as state and federal laws and Leapfrog, promote and mandate safe practices to improve patient safety and provide optimal, cost-effective care.
- **Accreditation agencies** provide mandates and standards for healthcare organizations and their leaders to reduce risk and improve patient safety. For example, the Joint Commission issued the National Patient Safety Goals (NPSGs) and the National Performance Goals (NPGs) to assist healthcare organizations in assessing and developing safe practices.
- **Professional organizations**, such as the American Medical Association and the American Nurses Association, have principles and codes of ethics that require quality care and patient safety.

EFFECT OF LEADERSHIP ON THE CULTURE OF SAFETY

Leadership is absolutely essential for developing the organization's patient safety culture because substantive change requires commitment from leadership to support the ideals of patient safety and provide the resources necessary to assess, train staff, and institute performance improvement methods to effect change. Leaders at all levels, from the governing board to the unit or department head, must work together to create a climate in which safety is expected as a first priority. Leadership must:

- **Model safe practices**: Leaders must consistently consider and demonstrate safe practices as part of their functions.
- **Preach safe practices**: Leaders must consistently address the need for safe practices and must provide information in support of patient safety.
- **Facilitate safe practices**: Leaders must provide training, education, equipment, staff, and other resources necessary to establish a culture of safety within the organization.

EFFECT OF MEDICAL ERRORS ON THE CULTURE OF SAFETY

Every assessment for patient safety culture must include a review of medical errors, which are unintentional but preventable mistakes in providing care. An error is a failure to carry out a planned action or a failure to use the correct plan. Adverse events are the negative results of errors, such as injuries and deaths.

- Errors may result from **commission** (doing something) or **omission** (failing to do something).
- Errors can be **active**, resulting from contact between the patient and an aspect of the medical system, such as a nurse or piece of equipment.
- Errors can be **latent**, resulting from a failure of system design.
- Error **chains** are the series of events that lead to a negative outcome, usually identified through root cause analysis.

Medical errors are most often identified after an adverse event occurs. Some go unidentified until they are found during medical record reviews. Typical errors include incorrect diagnoses, medication mistakes (such as wrong medication or dose), delays in reporting results, communication failure, improper or inadequate care, and mistaken identity.

EFFECT OF DIVERSITY ISSUES ON THE CULTURE OF SAFETY

Account for diversity when establishing a patient safety culture. Differences related to ethnic, religious, and cultural backgrounds might be easier to deal with than more institutionalized differences. Despite the best efforts of interdisciplinary teams and leadership, resistant subgroups of employees exist, such as those working in isolated areas, or those with a shared purpose or function, including such disparate groups as administrators, laboratory technicians, and housekeepers. Each group has its own perspective that must be respected. For example, within the organization there may be considerable differences in goals and perceptions between administrators and staff, and between doctors and nurses. Employees are often anxious regarding change and fear a loss of autonomy in working toward shared patient safety goals. Employees at all levels of the organization must be actively engaged in establishing a patient safety culture.

Safety Concepts

PATIENT SAFETY OFFICER

Effective patient safety programs need a full-time patient safety officer, trained and responsible for safety activities as their only occupation. The position should be one of high rank within the organization and invested with authority to make decisions and change processes to ensure safety. Responsibilities are to:

- Act as liaison officer for issues related to safety at all levels of the organization, and external agencies and organizations.
- Coordinate education and training activities and make safety presentations.
- Organize and coordinate with patient safety teams and other teams related to safety improvement.
- Provide periodic reviews and revisions of policies.
- Disseminate patient safety information and facilitate organization-wide communication.
- Establish a computerized error reporting system focused on process rather than individuals and punitive actions.
- Review medical error information, including trends and patterns.
- Establish rapid response teams and investigation processes.
- Complete risk assessment and risk management procedures.
- Facilitate performance measurement and staff incentive programs.

NCQA GUIDELINES

The National Committee for Quality Assurance (NCQA) addresses safety issues as part of its accreditation standards, in response to the Institute of Medicine's (IOM) call for accrediting agencies to ensure organizations focus on patient safety. Guidelines directed at managed care organizations provide useful information for all other organizations:

- Educate staff regarding clinical safety by providing information.
- Provide collaborative training within the network related to safe clinical practice.
- Combine data within the network [organization] on adverse outcomes/polypharmacy.
- Make improving patient safety a priority for quality improvement activities.
- Provide and distribute information about safe practices that includes information about computerized pharmacy order systems, intensive care-trained physicians, best practices, research on safe clinical practices.

JOINT COMMISSION'S NATIONAL PERFORMANCE GOALS

The Joint Commission published the National Performance Goals (NPGs) for hospitals in 2026 (replacing the previously used National Patient Safety Goals), intended to improve patient safety and efficiency of care in the inpatient setting. While the NPSGs are still in use for outpatient programs and include focuses on patient identification, medication safety, infection prevention, and preventing mistakes in surgery, the NPGs are targeted at the hospital setting and consist of 14 goals related to the following:

- Right patient, right care (The correct patient receives the correct care at the correct time.)
- Fostering a culture of safety
- Employing an emergency management program
- Prioritizing excellent health outcomes for all
- Prioritizing infection prevention and control

- Prioritizing pain management and safe prescribing
- Respecting the patient's right to safe and informed care
- Reducing the risk of suicide
- Implementing safe transplant practices
- Performing waived tests in a safe and consistent manner
- Maintaining workplace and patient safety
- Providing adequate staffing to meet the needs of the patients
- Practicing safe imaging services
- Employing a medication management program

APPLYING THE JOINT COMMISSION'S SAFETY GOALS TO AN ORGANIZATION

The Joint Commission (TJC) issues the National Performance Goals (NPGs) and the National Patient Safety Goals (NPSGs) under advisement of national experts. Goals and implementation expectations are listed for various types of programs. NPSGs are aimed at ambulatory care, assisted living, behavioral health care, disease-specific care, home care, laboratory, long-term care, networks, and office-based surgery. The NPGs are aimed at hospitals and critical-access hospitals, The CPHQ must identify those goals that apply to the organization. For example, the organization may have to comply with multiple safety standards related to ambulatory care, specific diseases, behavioral health, and laboratory programs.

Each year the NPSGs are updated (while the NPGs are only updated as evidence recommends). The organization must meet only those requirements that apply to the services it provides, and can bypass irrelevant requirements. The organization is responsible for compliance with NPG/NPSG requirements by staff, those granted privileges, and those with whom the organization has a contractual agreement.

Leadership must establish high priority for compliance with safety goals and ensure that the organization is at 90% compliance throughout the 12-month period before resurvey. This may require redefining patient care and development of new processes. Those who are noncompliant receive an RFI (requirement for improvement), which is used as part of the accreditation survey, so internal measurement and assessment must be conducted. Compliance with NPG/NPSG requirements is made public. New requirements may have a phase-in period, with testing at 3, 6, and 9 months, and implementation rules must be followed carefully.

JOINT COMMISSION INTERNATIONAL

The Joint Commission International (JCI) is a division of the Joint Commission Resources (JCR), the non-profit affiliate of the Joint Commission. The JCI provides international accreditation for safety and quality care for many types of healthcare organizations. The JCI provides internet-based self-assessment resources through the JCI Navigator, to assist organizations to manage quality and to achieve compliance with standards. International organizations can benefit from accreditation because it provides evaluation and goals for improvement and establishes that the organization complies with international safety standards. JCI provides measurements for benchmarking and risk reduction strategies. Individuals and some insurance companies are looking at JCI-accredited international organizations that provide more cost-effective healthcare than the US. The JCI process is designed with country-specific accommodations related to laws, religion, and culture.

JCI'S INTERNATIONAL PATIENT SAFETY GOALS

International healthcare organizations vary widely in their quality of care and attention to patient safety, depending on resources, training, national regulations, and standards. However, organizations accredited by the Joint Commission International can begin by focusing on integrating the **International Patient Safety Goals** through intensive staff education programs and monitoring for compliance:

- **Identify patients correctly**: Use two identifiers for medicines, blood, or blood products.
- **Improve effective communication**: Establish a process for taking orders and reports. Read back verbal and telephone orders.
- **Improve the safety of high-alert medications**.
- **Ensure safe surgery**: Utilize surgical checklists to confirm the correct patient, procedure, and body part. Ensure proper documentation and the necessary equipment is in working order. Mark surgical sites with clear, identifiable markings.
- **Reduce the risk of healthcare-associated infections**: Comply with hand washing standards according to the CDC guidelines.
- **Reduce the risk of patient harm resulting from falls**: Assess risk of falls and eliminate risks.

NATIONAL QUALITY FORUM

The National Quality Forum (NQF) is a non-profit membership organization for healthcare organizations interested in quality measurement and reporting to ensure better outcomes and patient safety. The goal of NQF is to promote national priorities for performance measurement and public reporting, working in collaboration with other agencies and partners to reach consensus on a core set of measures. Membership is granted to organizations, rather than individuals, so the governing board and administration must determine if they want to participate at a national level in establishing guidelines. Member organizations can participate in the national dialogue and can participate in the forum through membership in one of the main member councils: Consumer, Purchaser, Health Professional, Provider and Health Plan, and Research and Quality Improvement. NQF provides valuable educational forums and publications for member organizations related to factors in quality improvement, such as reporting and consideration of environmental factors.

According to NQF, the four elements needed to create and sustain a patient safety culture are:

- Leadership must ensure structures are in place for organization-wide awareness and compliance with safety measures, including adequate resources and direct accountability.
- Measurement, analysis, and feedback must track safety and allow for interventions.
- Team-based patient care with adequate training and performance improvement activities must be organization-wide.
- Safety risks must be continuously identified and interventions taken to reduce patient risk.

NQF SAFE PRACTICES

The National Quality Forum (NQF) endorses a set of safe practices to assess and develop an organization's patient safety culture. The NQF Safe Practices include:

- Considering the rights and responsibilities of the patient, providing informed consent, respecting advance directives and patient's directions related to care, and providing full disclosure of medical error.
- Providing adequate, well-trained, and supervised staff and resources to meet healthcare needs, and critical care-certified physicians for ICU or CCU.
- Managing information and care through proper documentation, providing prompt and accurate test results, utilizing standardized procedures for labeling diagnostic studies, and providing discharge planning.

- Managing medications by implementing a computerized prescriber order entry (CPOE) system, standardizing abbreviations, maintaining updated medication lists for patients, including pharmacists in medication management and selecting a formulary, standardizing labeling, identifying high alert drugs, and dispensing drugs in unit doses.
- Preventing healthcare-associated infections through ventilator bundle intervention, following best practices for central venous lines, complying with CDC hand washing guidelines, immunizing staff and patients for influenza, preventing surgical site infections through the appropriate use of antibiotics, mandating proper hair removal, reinforcing glucose control for cardiac patients, and maintaining temperature control for colorectal surgery.
- Providing safe practices for surgery, informing patients of risks, taking measures to prevent errors such as operating on the wrong site, and using prophylactic treatments as indicated to prevent complications.
- Providing procedures and ongoing assessment to prevent site-specific or treatment-specific adverse events, such as pressure ulcers, thromboembolism, deep vein thrombosis, allergic reactions, or anticoagulation complications.

INSTITUTE FOR HEALTHCARE IMPROVEMENT

The Institute for Healthcare Improvement (IHI) is a non-profit organization whose goal is to improve healthcare throughout the world through a focus on five key areas:

- Improvement capability
- Person- and family-centered care
- Patient safety
- Quality, cost, and value
- Quadruple Aim

IHI provides both free and fee-based programs and services. IHI launched healthcare initiatives, and offers books, videos, and audiotapes to provide guidance in quality improvement. IHI produces a series of free white papers, such as "Leadership Guide to Patient Safety," which outlines the eight steps an organization can follow to achieve patient safety. Much of the information provided by IHI is available free, including interactive tools for measuring adverse drug events and FMEA tools. IHI offers collaborative programs, such as the IMPACT Network, where organizations work together to facilitate changes at the system level, and Innovation Communities, which are collaborative learning laboratories. The patient safety guidelines cover broad areas and many apply to almost all healthcare organizations.

IHI 100,000 LIVES CAMPAIGN AND 5 MILLION LIVES CAMPAIGN

The IHI originally instituted a 100,000 lives campaign, with over 3,000 hospitals participating over an 18-month period. The campaign was focused on implementing six interventions to help avoid preventable loss of life:

- Deploy rapid response teams
- Deliver reliable, evidence-based care for acute MI
- Prevent adverse drug events
- Prevent central line infections
- Prevent surgical site infections
- Prevent ventilator-associated pneumonia

The **5 Million Lives Campaign** involved over 4,000 hospitals implementing twelve interventions this time over a 24-month period. The interventions included all six from the previous campaign while adding these six:

- Prevent harm from high alert medications
- Reduce surgical complications
- To prevent pressure ulcers
- Reduce methicillin-resistant *Staphylococcus aureus* (MRSA) infections
- Deliver reliable, evidence-based care for congestive heart failure to avoid readmissions
- Get boards on board to accelerate organizational progress toward safe care

INTEGRATING IHI PATIENT SAFETY GOALS INTO ORGANIZATIONAL ACTIVITIES

Information from IHI related to patient safety goals can be easily integrated into organizational activities. Members can participate in conferences, seminars, and internet-based programs. Materials can be utilized for training purposes as guidelines are based on best practices that readily apply to healthcare organizations. **Materials** that are available include:

- Guides to improvement in specific areas, such as decreasing ventilator-associated infections
- Evidence-based processes for change
- Tools, such as protocols, forms, and guidelines
- Links to internet resources
- Literature reviews

Because much of the information is free and downloadable from the IHI website, material specific to the needs of the organization can be included in education and training and used for integration of safety goals.

AHRQ QUALITY INDICATORS

The Agency for Healthcare Research and Quality (AHRQ) has developed Patient Safety Indicators (sets of specific quality indicators), regarding the potential for complications and adverse events for patients receiving treatment. AHRQ has sponsored the development of surveys for the assessment of patient safety for different healthcare organizations, including hospitals, nursing homes and outpatient facilities, and provides free software to allow the organization to compute its AHRQ quality improvement rate. Patient safety indicators are as follows:

- **Provider-level indicators**: Death rates (in low-mortality diagnosis related groups and in surgical inpatients with serious but treatable conditions), pressure ulcer rates, retained surgical items, iatrogenic pneumothorax rates, CLABSI rates, postoperative hip fracture rates, perioperative hematoma/hemorrhage rates, postoperative physiologic and metabolic derangement rate, postoperative PE/DVT rate, postoperative sepsis rate, transfusion reaction count, accidental puncture/laceration rate, and obstetric trauma rates.
- **Area-level indicators**: Retained surgical item rates, iatrogenic pneumothorax rates, CLABSI rates, postoperative wound dehiscence rates, accidental puncture/laceration rates, transfusion reaction rates, and postoperative hemorrhage/hematoma rates.

Some of the indicators are identified as both provider- and area-level indicators.

Hospitals may participate in data collection for research. For example, those participating in data collection regarding rates of CLABSI submitted data for entry into the AHRQ database each month directly or through the CDC's National Healthcare Safety Network (NHSN).

AHRQ Quality Indicators are distributed as a software tool free of charge to healthcare organizations to help them to identify adverse events or potential adverse events that require further study. This software is invaluable in developing an organization's patient safety culture. **Inpatient quality indicators for 2020** include the following:

Esophageal Resection Mortality Rate	Pancreatic Resection Mortality Rate	Abdominal Aortic Aneurysm Repair Mortality Rate
Coronary Artery Bypass Graft Mortality Rate	Acute Myocardial Infarction Mortality Rate	Heart Failure Mortality Rate
Acute Stroke Mortality Rate	Gastrointestinal Hemorrhage Mortality Rate	Hip Fracture Mortality Rate
Pneumonia Mortality Rate	Cesarean Delivery Rate, Uncomplicated	Vaginal Birth After Cesarean Delivery Rate, Uncomplicated
Percutaneous Coronary Intervention Mortality Rate	Carotid Endarterectomy Mortality	Laparoscopic Cholecystectomy rate
Primary Cesarean Delivery Rate, Uncomplicated	Vaginal Birth After Cesarean Rate, Uncomplicated	
Mortality for Selected Procedures	Mortality for Selected Conditions	

LEAPFROG

Leapfrog is a consortium of healthcare purchasers and employers that benefits millions of Americans. Leapfrog's initial focus was on reducing healthcare costs by preventing medical errors and "leaping forward" by rewarding hospitals and healthcare organizations that improve safety and quality of care. Leapfrog developed initiatives, based on the National Quality Forum's safety practices, to improve safety, which can be valuable tools for assessing and developing a patient safety culture. Leapfrog provides an annual **Hospital and Quality Safety Survey** to assess progress. It releases regional data and encourages voluntary public reporting. Leapfrog instituted the Leapfrog Hospital Rewards Program (LHRP) as a pay-for-performance program to reward organizations for showing improvement in key measures. Leapfrog promotes healthcare safety by focusing on "4 leaps" for hospitals to drive quality and patient safety:

- Computerized physician order entry (CPOE)
- Evidence-based hospital referrals
- ICU physician staffing
- Safe practices score

Leapfrog's **Safe Practices** include the following:

Culture of Safety Leadership Structures and Systems	Pharmacist Leadership Structures and Systems	Teamwork Training and Skill Building	Risks and Hazards	Informed consent	Life-Sustaining Treatment
Culture Measurement, Feedback, and Intervention	Multidrug-Resistant Organism Prevention	Venous Thromboembolism Prevention	Direct Caregivers	Intensive Care Unit Care	Patient Care Information
Order Read-Back and Abbreviations	Labeling Diagnostic Studies	Discharge Systems	Safe Adaptation of CPOE	Medication Reconciliation	Care of the Caregiver
Contrast Media-Induced Renal Failure Prevention	Catheter-Associated UTI Prevention	Daily Care of the Ventilated Patient	Surgical-Site Infection Prevention	Influenza Prevention	Hand Hygiene
Wrong-Site, Wrong-Procedure, Wrong-Person Surgery Prevention	Central Line-Associated Bloodstream Infection Prevention	Pressure Ulcer Prevention	Nursing Workforce	Disclosure	Organ Donation
Anticoagulation Therapy	Glycemic Control	Falls Prevention	Pediatric Imaging		

NATIONAL HEALTHCARE SAFETY NETWORK

The National Healthcare Safety Network (NHSN) integrates and replaces three separate programs: National Nosocomial Infections Surveillance (NNIS), Dialysis Surveillance Network (DSN), and National Surveillance System for Health Care Workers (NaSH). Participating in this program provides valuable **comparative data**. All healthcare facilities, such as hospitals and dialysis centers, can participate in the internet-based program that allows for reporting and sharing data. Those who apply to become members must agree to utilize CDC definitions, follow strict protocols, and submit data every six months. Anonymity of the institutions is protected. The program streamlines reporting of data and provides comparative data from across the United States. The system can identify sentinel or unusual events and notify appropriate participating agencies. There are three components to NHSN: Patient safety, healthcare worker safety, and research and development. Extensive data analysis features are part of the program. Reports of nosocomial, or hospital-acquired, infections that were previously issued by NNIS are now issued by NHSN.

DEVELOPING PATIENT SAFETY PROGRAMS

Each healthcare organization has unique needs and challenges to face in developing a patient safety program, although many components are universally needed. Facilitating development of a patient safety program requires planning and taking these steps:

- Identify a quality professional or interdisciplinary group to manage the safety program.
- Define the scope of the program, including risk identification, management, and response to adverse events.

- Provide mechanisms to integrate all aspects of the program into organization-wide functions.
- Establish procedures for rapid response to medical errors or adverse events.
- Establish procedures for both internal and external reporting of medical errors.
- Define and disseminate intervention strategies, such as risk reduction, risk tracking, and root cause analysis.
- Outline mechanisms for staff support related to involvement in sentinel events.
- Establish procedures and responsibilities for reporting to the governing board.

A patient safety program must include these components:

- Functional infrastructure with leader, safety officer, teams, and software for tracking and measures.
- Linkage of program goals with strategic goals of the organization.
- Establishment of policies and procedures to reduce and control risk, and supportive training.
- Reporting system to identify adverse events or incidents.
- Participation in national patient safety initiatives, such as NPSG, NPG, IPSG, IHI 5 Million Lives, and Leapfrog.
- Rapid response procedures to deal with medical errors and sentinel events.
- Adequate data collection procedures to ensure performance measurement, tracking, and data analysis.
- Performance improvement activities directed at specific goals.
- Documentation of all processes, procedures, reporting, and timelines.

PHYSICIAN PARTICIPATION IN A PATIENT SAFETY PROGRAM

Physician participation is a necessary component of any patient safety program. Physicians must be active partners in the organization's methods to reduce patient risk and improve risk management. Doctors, like other health professionals, are concerned that error reports are kept confidential and non-discoverable, and that evidence is used to improve processes, rather than for punitive actions. Involve physicians in the following:

- Identifying areas of potential risks in patient care processes.
- Designing risk reduction programs for clinical care.
- Developing criteria for identifying potential or actual clinical risk cases.
- Evaluating specific cases that have been identified as having risks.
- Actively participating in process improvement teams and risk management to promote patient safety and correct problems.

Environmental Considerations in a Patient Safety Program

Steps to evaluate environmental safety hazards and risks for a safety program are as follows:

1. Prepare a written plan that clearly outlines environmental safety concerns, policies, and procedures.
2. Establish a safe environment for staff and patients, including fall prevention strategies, such as installing handrails, contrast strips on stairways, and analyzing work flow to facilitate functions.
3. Identify security risks, such as infant/child abduction, and establish processes to increase security, such as alarms, ID badges, locks, better lighting, and security officers.
4. Follow EPA and state regulations and educate staff about correct identification, handling, storage, and disposal of hazardous wastes, including corrosives, flammables, reactives, and toxics.
5. Conduct fire safety drills and check equipment and buildings for fire dangers.
6. Monitor medical equipment, ensuring routine maintenance, testing and regular inspection.
7. Evaluate power/utility requirements, including emergency power, and maintain, test, and inspect utilities.
8. Designate individuals to monitor and coordinate environmental safety management and to develop procedures for dealing with threats/problems.
9. Complete a risk assessment of the physical plant, including buildings, grounds, equipment, and related systems, such as electrical, lighting, IT, ventilation, and plumbing.
10. Establish organization-wide safety policies and procedures, including no smoking policies.
11. Maintain the physical plant by monitoring and responding to product recalls.
12. Establish a plan for emergency preparedness; evaluate areas of vulnerability, test preparedness, response, and recovery times.
13. Establish an interdisciplinary team to identify opportunities for improvement and facilitate performance improvement processes.

Incorporating Systems and Individuals in a Patient Safety Program

When developing a patient safety program, consider the errors that relate to systems and those that relate to individuals in the program design:

- **Systems**: Most errors are related to inefficient or flawed systems, rather than individual error. Systems errors are the consequence of systemic deficiencies, such as inadequate staffing, insufficient third-party payments, poor maintenance, and outdated equipment, policies, and procedures. Some of these factors are internal, but others are external, so the organization has little control over them. Mitigate these factors as much as possible to improve safety.
- **Individuals**: Humans make mistakes despite the best planning and systems, so plan ways to immediately identify and decrease errors, such as through computerized physician order entry (CPOE), bar coding, and triggers for data collection that allow for identification of errors so the effects are mitigated.

EVIDENCE-BASED PRACTICE

Use evidence-based practice (EBP) for integrating safety concepts into an organization. EBP is based on the best available scientific and clinical information, characterized as "best practices." Although information about best practices is readily available, the best quality care is not always provided. Two examples of adverse events caused by ignoring EBP are:

- Failure to give Aspirin to a patient in the emergency room with a possible myocardial infarction, leading to blood clots.
- Treating a viral infection with antibiotics, which is inappropriate and of little value.

Utilizing EBP ensures that practitioners are aware of best practices and that systems are set up in such a way to influence their decision-making, such as through the use of:

- Clinical decision support system (CDSS).
- Computerized physician/provider order entry (CPOE).
- Establishing protocols and standing orders.

INTEGRATING QUALITY MANAGEMENT INTO PATIENT SAFETY CONCEPTS

Organizations that have already instituted a program of quality management, such as continuous quality improvement (CQI) or total quality management (TQM), are in a good position to integrate patient safety concepts within their organizations. The goal of quality management is to look at processes at all levels of an organization, identify opportunities for improvement, and institute change. Data collection, measurement, and analysis are already institutionalized, so the primary change is that the concept of patient safety must be identified as a high priority goal of quality management. Focus efforts on improving safety by using guides such as the National Patient Safety Goals (NPSGs) and National Performance Goals (NPGs). Safety concepts are then automatically integrated through the assessment and performance improvement process.

SAFETY BY-LAWS, ADMINISTRATIVE POLICIES, AND PROCEDURES

Integrating patient safety findings into governance and management activities establishes the organization's commitment to patient safety.

- The **by-laws** should specify lines of authority and responsibility at all levels in the organization related to patient safety.
- The **governing board** establishes the method by which safety issues are reported, and this should include the designated person to report, a specific timeline, and reporting requirements.
- Patient safety responsibilities, which are based on patient safety findings, should be included in **job descriptions** and should be delineated as part of administrative policies and duties.
- **Administrative policies** must emphasize all departments and areas of the organization are required to participate in safety activities and respond to patient safety findings.

Evaluate all existing procedures and processes organization-wide, revise them as necessary, and institute new procedures in response to findings.

DEVELOPING AND REVISING WRITTEN HOSPITAL SAFETY PLANS

The hospital safety plan is a major component in the quality improvement plan for the organization, which ensures safety concerns are integrated into assessment and action plans. However, the safety plan should focus directly on the organization's commitment to providing a safe environment. Include an **introductory section** that references the mission or vision statement of the organization, outlining how the safety plan relates to the strategic goals.

Next, explain the scope of the plan:

1. A statement of purpose that explains the main focus of the plan, such as "reduce mortality" or "improve patient care by identifying risks"
2. Specific goals, objectives, or priorities in performance improvement activities related to safety, with the steps to achieving these outlined
3. An explanation of responsibilities, including those of the governing board, safety officer, staff members, patients, visitors, and volunteers
4. An explanation of confidentiality
5. A plan for evaluation

MEDICATION SAFETY

According to a 2020 study conducted by the Yale School of Medicine, about 7,000 deaths of previously healthy individuals each year in the United States are attributed to **medication errors**. Ensure patient safety with proper handling and administration of medications:

- **Avoid error-prone abbreviations or symbols**. The Joint Commission has established a list of abbreviations to avoid, but mistakes are frequent with other abbreviations, too. Avoid abbreviations and symbols altogether, or restrict them to a limited, approved list.
- **Prevent errors from illegible handwriting**. Enter orders into a computer program. Handwritten orders should be block printed to reduce errors.
- Institute bar coding and scanners that allow the patient's wristband and medication to be scanned for verification.
- Provide lists of **similarly-named and look-alike medications** to educate staff.
- **Establish an institutional policy** for administering medications that includes protocols for verification of drug, dosage, time, and patient identification. Educate the patient about his or her medications.

ERRORS IN PATIENT SAFETY

Thousands of patients die each year in hospitals because of errors in patient safety, with estimates ranging from the tens of thousands to the hundreds of thousands. A caring environment must be a safe environment for patients and their families. Patient safety is impacted by these factors:

- **Staffing practices**: Patient-staff ratios are of primary importance, as having fewer staff working longer hours results in more errors. This is especially true in critical care areas, such as NICU or PICU. The expertise of the staff is another important factor. An increased proportion of care by registered nurses decreases both hospital stay and complications.
- **Infection control**: The rates of hospital infections have steadily increased because of antibiotic-resistant pathogens (such as *Staphylococcus aureus* and MRSA) that are now endemic in some institutions. Patients with invasive devices, such as central lines or ventilators, are at increased risk. Much infection is related to poor hand washing and infection control practices on the part of staff.

Hand Disinfection
CDC's Hand Washing Guidelines
All patients are potentially infectious, so staff must wash their hands before and after every direct contact with a patient or when removing gloves. Hand contamination is one of the most common causes of person-to-person transmission of infection. Train all medical personnel in hand washing techniques and observe them regularly for compliance. The CDC's recommended procedure is reproduced below:

- Hands should be washed using soap and warm, running water.
- Hands should be rubbed vigorously during washing for at least 20 seconds with special attention paid to the backs of the hands, wrists, between the fingers and under the fingernails.
- Hands should be rinsed well while leaving the water running.
- With the water running, hands should be dried with a single-use towel.
- Turn off the water using a paper towel, covering washed hands to prevent re-contamination.

Alcohol-Based Rubs
While soap and water hand washing has been the standard for many years, alcohol-based rubs used correctly, of adequate concentration, kill twice as much bacteria in the same amount of time. Alcohol rubs are less irritating to the hands than repeated washing. Staff must be trained in use and observed for compliance. Hand fires have occurred when staff members smoke with alcohol-wet hands. Sample procedure:

- Hand disinfection is done for at least 15 seconds by using an alcohol-based rub and should be done before and after contact with a patient or after removal of gloves.
- All hand surfaces should be thoroughly coated with the alcohol-rub, including between the fingers, the wrists, and under the nails, and then the hands rubbed together until the solution evaporates.
- Hands should not be rinsed.
- Alcohol-based rubs disinfect but do not mechanically clean hands, so hands that are dirty or contaminated should be washed first with soap and water.

Emergency Medical Treatment and Active Labor Act
The Emergency Medical Treatment and Active Labor Act (EMTALA) prevents patient "dumping" from emergency departments (ED) and concerns risk management, requiring staff training for compliance:

- Transfers from ED may be intrahospital or to another facility.
- Stabilization of the patient with emergency conditions or active labor must be done in the ED prior to transfer.
- Patient screening must be given prior to inquiring about insurance or the ability to pay.
- Stabilization requires treatment for emergency conditions and the doctor must have a reasonable belief that, although the emergency condition may not be completely resolved, the patient's condition will not deteriorate during transfer.
- Women in the ED in active labor should deliver both the child and placenta before transfer.

- The receiving department or facility should be capable of treating the patient and dealing with possible complications.
- Transfer to another facility is indicated if the patient requires specialized services not available intrahospital, such as to a burn center or NICU.

PROFESSIONAL LIABILITY

Risk managers must define professional liability for staff and ensure that related risks are minimized. Direct care providers must obtain written consents for Medicare, provide adequate care, and obey drug laws.

- **Physicians are liable for**: Misdiagnoses, lack of staff supervision, providing incorrect or substandard treatment, treating patients outside their area of expertise, failing to provide follow-up care, failing to seek necessary consultation, infections resulting from procedures, premature discharge, and lack of proper documentation.
- **Nurses are liable for**: Improper administration of drugs; failing to follow standard medical procedures; failing to follow physicians' written orders; taking incorrect verbal orders; failing to report changes in patients' conditions or defective equipment; miscounting sponges, instruments, and surgical equipment; avoidable injuries to patients from falls or burns; and mishandling patients' personal belongings.

NEGLIGENCE

Risk managers must determine the burden of proof for acts of negligence, including compliance with duty, breaches in procedures, degree of harm, and cause. Negligence means proper care was not provided, based on established standards. Reasonable care uses rationales for decision-making in relation to providing care. State regulations regarding negligence vary, but all have some statutes of limitation. The **types of negligence** are:

- **Negligent conduct**, which indicates that an individual failed to provide reasonable care or failed to protect or assist another, based on standards and their level of expertise.
- **Gross negligence** is willfully providing inadequate care, while disregarding the safety and security of another.
- **Contributory negligence** involves the injured party contributing to his or her own harm (e.g., a drug addict who overdoses).
- **Comparative negligence** determines the percentage amount of negligence attributed to each individual involved.

> **Review Video: Medical Negligence**
> Visit mometrix.com/academy and enter code: 928405

LOSS AND RISK EXPOSURE

Risk management includes loss prevention, taking proactive measures to eliminate loss, and loss reduction, taking reactive measures to decrease potential loss. Risk managers must identify risk exposure through continuous data collection of occurrences or adverse events, including external review, patient complaints, financial audits, referrals, observations, contracts, current litigation, and risky practices. Continuous analysis must also be conducted in the following areas:

- **Liability**, including malpractice and defamation actions
- **Employer-related issues**, including Workers Compensation, hiring, terminating, intellectual property losses, and death or disability of employees

- **Property and environment issues**, including injuries related to equipment or physical plant, chemical or nuclear wastes, and transportation vehicles
- **Financial or contract issues**, including embezzlement, theft, anti-trust actions related to peer review, contracts, fraud and abuse, and securities violations

Risk Avoidance and Prevention

Risk management aligns with quality management in determining measures for risk avoidance and prevention. In the analysis process, adverse events may be shown to relate to dysfunction in the organization, increasing risk exposure, so risk managers must make efforts to decrease this exposure:

- **Financial management** includes determining both risk retention and risk transfer:
  - **Risk retention** occurs when the organization assumes financial responsibility for risks.
  - **Risk transfer** occurs when financial responsibility for risks is transferred to an insurance company through policies.
- **Risk event control** involves development of specific programs and processes to limit risk exposure:
  - **Avoidance** eliminates that which causes risk, such as a particularly high-risk neonatal program.
  - **Shifting** changes internal responsibility for risk to external through contract services or referrals.
  - **Prevention** changes processes to reduce adverse events, such as using disposable equipment to reduce infection rates.

Claims Management

Risk management involves administrative functions like claims management and taking action on potentially compensable events (PCE), those liability events that may incur costs to the organization. The steps for claims management are:

1. **Plan ahead**: The organization must be prepared with a plan to deal with different types of PCE, such as disability claims.
2. **Evaluation**: A complete examination of the incident/claim should be undertaken as soon as possible to gather information, to determine liability, and decide whether it would be cost-effective to offer a settlement.
3. **Document carefully**: Proper documentation must be a continuous, proactive process, rather than reactive.
4. **Consult with insurance companies/Workman's Compensation and legal experts**: Provide information to assist insurers to make decisions about claims and retain legal assistance as needed.
5. **Provide support and assistance**: Being responsive to the needs of claimants may avoid a liability suit.
6. **Maintain financial records**: Carefully maintain records of claims management costs.

Safety Principles

INNOVATIVE SYSTEMS THINKING AND RESOURCE USE

Innovative systems thinking and resource use among the healthcare team requires empowering staff to make decisions and to identify needs that require resource allocations. Administration must look for nursing leaders who are open to nontraditional methods and not afraid to change. Consider the Star Model, based on a star diagram, in which the points are: Strategy, Structure, Human Resources, Incentives, Information and Decision-making. Star has a core of systemic culture and values:

- Staff laziness or inability is rarely the root cause of systemic problems.
- There is more than one optimal system, depending on internal and external factors.
- One point is not more important than another.
- A change in one area usually necessitates a change in another.
- The culture and values cannot be changed directly, but only indirectly through action on one of the points.
- Ingrained cultures and values can impede progress.

STEPS TO SYSTEMS THINKING

Systems thinking is a critical thinking approach to problem solving that takes an organization-wide perspective to address errors. This is a shift from traditional thinking where an individual is considered the source of error. Systems thinking considers all aspects of a process and the potential implications for a broader approach. Introduce systems thinking when there is a lack of consensus, effective change is stalemated, and standards are inconsistent. Follow these steps:

- **Define the issue**: Describe the problem in detail. Do not judge or offer solutions.
- **Describe behavior patterns**: List factors related to the problem. Use graphs to outline possible trends.
- **Establish cause-effect relationships**: Use the Five Whys or another root cause analysis method, or feedback loops.
- **Define patterns of performance/behavior**: Determine how variables affect outcomes and the types of patterns of behavior currently taking place.
- **Find solutions**: Discuss possible solutions and outcomes.
- **Institute performance improvement activities**: Make process changes and then monitor for changes in behavior.

PROMOTING ORGANIZATIONAL VALUES AND COMMITMENT

Systems thinking focuses on how systems interrelate, with each part affecting the entire system. For the CPHQ to promote organizational values and commitment, the organization must embrace systems thinking and its associated concepts:

- **Individual responsibility**: Encourage individual workers to establish their own goals within the organization and to work toward a purpose.
- **Learning process**: Respect the internalized beliefs of the staff and build upon these beliefs to establish a mindset based on continuous learning and improvement.
- **Vision**: Share the organizational vision to help staff understand the purpose of change and to build commitment.
- **Team process**: Assist teams to develop good listening and collaborative skills, so dialog increases and they are able to reach consensus.
- **Systems thinking**: Encourage staff members to understand the interrelationship of all members of the organization and to appreciate how any change affects the whole.

CONSIDERING PATIENT CHARACTERISTICS

The synergy method for patient care recognizes that there are a number of patient characteristics that must be considered when matching a staff member's competencies to the needs of the patient and his or her family:

- **Resiliency** is the ability to recover from a devastating illness and regain a sense of stability, both physically and emotionally. Things that support resiliency are faith, a positive sense of hope, and a supportive network of friends and family.
- **Vulnerability** means the patient is susceptible to infection; has increased risk for disease; recovery is slowed; or is non-compliant because of anxiety, fear, lack of support, chronic illness, prejudice, and lack of information.
- **Stability** allows a patient and family to maintain a state of physical and/or emotional equilibrium despite illness and challenges. Important factors include: Relief from stress, conflicts, or emotional burdens; motivation; and values.
- **Complexity** occurs when more than one system is involved, and these can be internal (cardiac and renal systems) or external (addicted and homeless) or some combination (ill with poor family dynamics).

Human Factors Engineering

Human factors engineering is the discipline involved in trying to identify those things related to engineering, manufacturing, and human interaction that may lead to errors, such as two different medications that look alike or different manufacturers for the same type of equipment. Human factors engineering includes assessing tasks involved in processes, including the physical, skill, and knowledge requirements, as well as the environment (heat, light, distractions) and equipment design. A number of different approaches are utilized to address safety:

- **Testing usability**: Identifying "workarounds" that staff members develop to cope with poor design or practice in order to improve efficiency or save time but can lead to serious errors.
- **Forcing function**: Taking action that prevents an error or requiring a specific step before another can be performed.
- **Utilizing standardization**: Using checklists and standardized equipment and processes to prevent errors.
- **Evaluating resiliency**: Considering how the organization anticipates change/problems and handles them.

High-Reliability Organizations

High-reliability organizations are those that involve hazardous work or environments but have a lower-than-usual occurrence of adverse events. All healthcare organizations strive for high-reliability but errors and adverse events remain common. Principles of high-reliability organizations include:

- **Constant concern regarding failure**: The organization recognizes risks inherent in healthcare and is constantly on the alert for areas/situations that may produce errors and makes use of human factors engineering.
- **Focus on promoting resilience**: The organization responds quickly to problems/errors and has the ability to identify threats before they cause harm.
- **Attention to operations**: Healthcare workers report problems and unsafe conditions when they observe them and are provided some autonomy in dealing with problems and unsafe conditions.
- **Adequate communication**: Documentation standards are adhered to and handoff procedures are standardized.
- **Promotion of a culture of safety**: Safety is a concern at all levels in the organization and staff members are rewarded rather than intimidated for reporting safety concerns.
- **Reluctance to simplify**: The organization is thorough when identifying the root cause of a patient safety concern and avoids selecting the simplest answer to determine the reason for success or failure.
- **Deference to expertise**: The organization ensures that feedback is solicited from the individuals performing critical tasks on a daily basis to identify risks to patient safety.

Risk Management Programs

Risk management is an organized, formal method of decreasing liability, financial loss, and risk or harm to patients, staff, or others by assessment and strategies. Risk management is driven by the insurance industry to minimize costs, and by quality managers to ensure quality healthcare and process improvement. A **risk management program** usually has a manager and specially trained staff responsible for:

- **Risk identification**, which begins with an assessment of current processes to identify and prioritize those that require further study to determine risk exposure.
- **Risk analysis**, which requires careful documentation of the process through flow charts and root cause analysis, with each step in the process assessed for potential risks.
- **Risk prevention**, which involves identifying and training responsible teams to institute corrective or preventive processes.
- **Assessment and evaluation** of corrective and preventive processes are ongoing to determine if they are effective or require modification.

Enterprise risk management (ERM) is growing in popularity within the healthcare industry as organizations are tasked with considering risk far beyond clinical care to ensure longevity. Enterprise risk management is a holistic approach to identifying potential threats and developing processes and procedures to be positioned to address them effectively. ERM considers seven key areas to prepare for uncertainty: strategic, financial, legal/regulatory, operational, human capital, technology, and hazard.

EARLY WARNING SYSTEM

Risk management is concerned with decreasing liability and increasing safety. Integrating the outcomes of risk management assessment into the performance improvement process requires an organization-wide commitment to reducing risk. The governing board and CPHQ ensure that risk management assessments are considered when formulating mission and vision statements and strategic goals. Risk management assessment is one of the first concerns during process evaluation and process improvement. An **organization-wide early warning system** should be in place to screen patients for potential risks and identify:

- **Adverse patient occurrences (APOs)**, unexpected events that negatively impact the patient's health or welfare.
- **Potentially compensable events (PCEs),** which are APO's that may result in claims against the organization because of their negative impact on the patient's health or welfare.

If the organization has set up a method to quickly identify problems, then risks are minimized.

DEVELOPING OR REVISING WRITTEN PLANS FOR RISK MANAGEMENT PROGRAM

The written risk management plan, while not required by accreditation agencies, is usually required by liability insurers. The written plan must include:

- **Statement of purpose**: Outline the organization's general policy of risk management, such as patient safety guidelines or financial risk reductions.
- **Goals**: Make goals specific and measurable.
- **Program scope**: Include linkages with other programs.
- **Lines of authority**: Begin with the governing board and end with employees. Outline the responsibilities at each level.
- **Policies**: Include confidentiality (HIPAA) and conflict of interest policies.
- **Data sources and referrals**: Outline the types of measures the organization uses.
- **Documentation/reporting**: Clarify who is responsible for reporting. List the frequency of reports.
- **Evaluation of program**: Method and frequency of evaluation.
- **Charts and diagrams**: Attach flow charts, organizational charts, and pertinent diagrams to the written risk management plan.

Safety Reviews

ENSURING COMPLIANCE WITH SAFETY STANDARDS

The process of patient safety goals review is an important function to ensure that there is compliance with safety standards. A process may be chosen for review as part of regular monitoring or because outcomes show an opportunity for improvement. Determine the safety guidelines that will be used, for example, the Joint Commission's NPSG specific for hospitals. Perform interviews, observations, data collection and analysis. Identify and document how each safety guideline is implemented. For example, one safety guideline is to improve patient identification. Pose these questions to determine if this guideline is met:

- Does the patient wear an identification bracelet issued by Admitting?
- Does the provider check the bracelet?
- Does the provider ask for identifying information, such as birth dates?
- How consistently are these procedures followed?

MORTALITY REVIEWS

The risk of dying in a healthcare institution varies widely from one facility to another, with mortality rates twice as high in some institutions as in others; thus, mortality reviews are a critical element of risk management. Mortality reviews are conducted to determine if treatments and patient care were adequate and appropriate, and if any deaths were preventable, with the goal of reducing mortality. Mortality review includes mortality data and individual case review. When establishing a procedure for mortality review, select a timeframe or a specified number of consecutive deaths, and investigate all deaths that occurred during that timeframe or within that consecutive set. Mortality review steps are:

- Screen for deaths, manually or electronically.
- A non-physician team performs an initial analysis to determine if further evaluation is needed or if each death was unavoidable.
- Physicians review the avoidable cases for medical management, and a multidisciplinary team reviews them for patient care processes.
- A final peer review is conducted by physicians, departments and management for process and root cause analyses.

ROLE IN QUALITY MANAGEMENT

The mortality review is an important tool for quality management because it presents quantifiable information that provides opportunities for improvement. Mortality reviews include not only the organization's total death rate but also department-level death rates, and these are compared with external data. When reviewing mortality rates and targeting areas for improvement, consider the number of:

- Patients who were poor surgical risks.
- Deaths in the emergency department.
- Patients with "do not resuscitate" (DNR) orders.
- Patients who were terminal on admission.
- Patients whose hospital stays were lengthened rather than being transferred to extended care facilities.
- Deaths attributed to hospital-acquired and community-acquired infections.
- Patterns of death by department or physician that suggest poor quality care or negligence.

- Patients referred for peer review before and after the mortality review.
- In-service education and training sessions.

Mortality Review and Measurement of Outcomes

Mortality review is an efficient measure of outcomes. When faced with the need for performance improvement organization-wide, quality professionals may have an enormous number of improvement opportunities, all requiring assessment, prioritizing, and plans, which is time-consuming and causes delays in improving processes, so mortality rates are a good beginning point for these reasons:

- Deaths must be recorded and reported with the cause of death, so data is readily available and easy to access.
- Deaths provide quantifiable data.
- Mortality rates are good indicators of overall quality performance.
- The mortality review helps to identify patterns and areas of concern within the organization.
- Because mortality reviews are retrospective, the search for information and records is simplified.
- Understanding the reason for mortality rates helps to establish performance improvement activities that directly target causes.

Integration of Risk Management with Quality Management

Risk management must integrate with quality management as part of process improvement. Risk management holds a central role in quality management because it focuses on achieving positive outcomes and reducing risks and liability. Both quality management and risk management share the commitment to providing optimal care and utilizing measurement and data regarding incidents, performance surveillance, root cause analysis, and feedback to evaluate, design, and monitor processes. Risk managers must be familiar with accreditation and state regulatory statutes in relation to both risk management and quality management. State regulations vary in regard to confidentiality and immunity, and in some states, documentation related to quality measures and risk concerns must be maintained separately. However, the Joint Commission's standards require that quality management and risk management be linked.

Activities Improving Patient Safety

Patient safety performance improvement activities are campaigns to reduce error or improve patient outcomes. For example, a campaign to reduce postoperative infections involves performance improvement activities for surgeons, O.R. staff, ward staff, housekeeping staff, Environmental Services, Infection Control, Microbiology, patients' families, and allied health workers. The scope could be limited to one type of patient — diabetic kidney/pancreas transplant patients, for example — or could be broader, involving all surgical patients for June–December. A multidisciplinary problem like this one may involve surveillance, new purchasing contracts, new vaccinations, translations, training, rescheduling workflow and worksites, and procedure modifications (e.g., monitoring air flow to negative-pressure rooms and placing hand antiseptics in every room). Performance and process improvement are central to the Joint Commission's accreditation standards. Begin by reading the standards to flag possible improvement activities. Next, look at the collected data that pertains to those flags. Teams must decide what to measure, how to collect data, brainstorm solutions, and then implement solutions in a concerted effort.

INCIDENT REPORT REVIEW

Incident report review is part of risk management because incidents represent a failure in the system. Incident reports may be filled out by individuals who are involved in the incident, or who observed the incident. Increasingly, incident reports are generated by electronic data that indicates an error occurred, such as in medication administration. Incident report reviews are less comprehensive and time-consuming and more cost-effective than retrospective medical record reviews but can yield valuable information. Provide staff with incentives for reporting and assure them that confidentiality will be maintained. Incidents are grossly underreported in healthcare organizations. Reviews help determine if incidents are being accurately reported, so patterns and trends are identified early. The CPHQ may interview physicians and staff. A review looks at the incident in terms of process steps and determines where in the process an error occurred in order to establish a plan for improvement.

SENTINEL EVENT REVIEW

Sentinel events are unexpected occurrences that result in death, significant morbidity, or the risk of either. These are "special cause" variations in the data, outside of normal variations, and must trigger further analysis if the event either occurred within an organization or was related to services provided by an organization. Review includes:

- Utilization of an established process for review of sentinel events.
- Completion of root cause analysis, which must include participation of leadership and all those involved in the process, and a review of standard practices and literature.
- Action plan formulated to reduce the risk of recurrence of the adverse event, indicating those responsible for implementing and monitoring the action plan.
- Timelines for compliance with action plans and outcomes.
- Training provided as necessary.
- Action plan piloted, modified as needed, implemented, and reviewed.
- Documentation of the complete sentinel event review process.

ROOT CAUSE ANALYSIS

Root cause analysis (RCA) is a retrospective attempt to determine the cause of a sentinel event, such as an unexpected death, or a cluster of events. Root cause analysis involves interviews, observations, and reviews of medical records. Often, an extensive questionnaire is completed by the professional doing the RCA, tracing essentially every step in the patient's hospitalization and care, including each treatment, each medication, and each contact. RCA focuses on systems and processes, rather than blaming individuals. How did the system break down? Where did the problem arise? In some cases, there may be one root cause, but in others, the causes may be multiple. The RCA must include a thorough literature review to ensure that process improvement plans based on the results of the RCA reflect current best practices. Plans without RCA are non-productive. If, for example, an infection is caused by contaminated air, process improvement plans to increase disinfection of the Operating Room surfaces would be ineffective.

Failure Mode and Effects Analysis (FMEA)

Failure mode and effects analysis (FMEA) is a team-based prospective analysis method that attempts to identify and correct failures in a process before utilization to ensure positive outcomes. The steps for FMEA are:

1. **Definition**: Describe the entire process and outline the scope of the FMEA.
2. **Team creation**: Assemble a temporary, interdisciplinary ad hoc team for a specific FMEA process, whose members are involved in the process or have the necessary expertise.
3. **Description**: Create a flow chart, number each step in the process consecutively, and letter each sub-step consecutively. Complex processes require focus and prioritizing. Generate a final, permanent document with all the steps.
4. **Brainstorming**: Discuss each step and sub-step for potential failure modes, considering major categories such as people, processes, equipment, and environment. Make an affinity diagram. Number and letter possible failures to correspond with the steps and sub-steps on the flow chart.
5. **Identify potential causes of potential failures**: Create a cause-and-effect diagram. Conduct root cause analysis or utilize Five Whys, and record potential causes on a worksheet.
6. **List potential adverse outcomes**: Identify the results of failures to the patient.
7. **Assign a severity rating**: Rate each potential adverse outcome (identified in step 6) on a scale of 1–10 for severity of the failure, with 1 being a slight annoyance and 10 being death.
8. **Assign an occurrence rating**: Rate each potential failure on a scale of 1–10, with 1 (remote) being a frequency of 1:10,000 and 10 (very high) being a frequency of 1:20, showing the probability of the failure occurring within a specified time period, usually a year.
9. **Assign a detection rating**: Rate each potential failure on a scale of 1–10 to determine the likelihood that hazards, errors, or failures will be identified prior to their occurrence. 10 (very high) is a near certainty that the errors will be detected. 1 (remote) is a 1/10 or less probability that errors will be detected.
10. **Calculate the Risk Priority Number (RPN)**: Calculate the criticality index to determine if tasks remain on the critical path with this formula:
    a. Take the results of all three scales from steps 7, 8 and 9 (i.e., **S**everity, **O**ccurrence, and **D**etection)
    b. Multiply (S × O × D) to find the RPN
11. **Reduce potential failures**: The team brainstorms control measures to reduce or eliminate potential failures and identifies where in the process to place control measures. A leader is assigned to monitor and pilot test the control measures.
12. **Identify performance measures**: Introduce measures to monitor the modified process and reduce the RPN.

Quality Review and Accountability

Standards and Best Practices

HEALTHCARE EFFECTIVENESS DATA AND INFORMATION SET (HEDIS)

The Healthcare Effectiveness Data and Information Set (HEDIS) is a tool utilized by greater than 90% of health plans to measure performance of over 90 measures in 6 domains of care:

- **Effectiveness of care** includes measures for which clinical standards of care exist, such as prevention and screening, diabetes, cardiovascular conditions, musculoskeletal conditions, respiratory conditions, behavioral health, and overuse/appropriate use.
- **Access/Availability of care** includes measures that track timely access to preventive and ambulatory health services, dental visits, and prenatal and postpartum care.
- **Experience of care** includes measures that assess perception of care.
- **Utilization and risk-adjusted utilization** includes measures related to antibiotic utilization, mental health utilization, hospitalizations, and readmissions.
- **Health plan descriptive information** includes details pertaining to the health plan product, such as the enrollment by product line or the number of board-certified providers that provide care to health plan members.
- **Measures reported using electronic clinical data systems** are data points from networks such as the EHR, Health Information Exchanges (HIEs), immunization registries, or other clinical registries that provide insight into a patient's experience. This information is transmitted to the health plan at a predetermined cadence to reduce the administrative burden of medical chart reviews and ensure accuracy and reliability of data for HEDIS reporting.

HEDIS data are collected from health plans and physicians and compiled in databases and can be used to compare health plan performance. HEDIS is updated annually by the National Committee for Quality Assurance (NCQA) with measures added, deleted, and revised. HEDIS data collection is through surveys, insurance claims and medical chart reviews and is mandated by CMS for Medicare Advantage HMO plans and by NCQA's accreditation process. Measures may apply to commercial health plans, Medicaid, and/or Medicare as appropriate. HEDIS data may be utilized to assess external best practices and the quality of performance, set performance goals, and identify cost-effective interventions.

> **Review Video: Medicare & Medicaid**
> Visit mometrix.com/academy and enter code: 507454

JOINT COMMISSION CORE MEASURES

The Joint Commission has established core measures to determine if healthcare institutions are in compliance with current standards. The core measures involve a series of questions that are answered either "yes" or "no" to indicate if an action was completed. Currently, the Joint Commission's core measures pertain to the following:

- Assisted Living Community
- Cardiac Care
- Emergency Department
- Healthcare Staffing Services
- Hospital Outpatient Department
- Hospital-Based Inpatient Psychiatric Services
- Immunization
- Palliative Care
- Perinatal Care
- Spine Surgery
- Stroke
- Substance Use
- Tobacco Treatment
- Total Hip and Knee Replacement
- Venous Thromboembolism

For each measure, questions relate to whether or not standard care was provided, such as giving an aspirin to patients with an acute MI. This data is public and provides useful information about these particular standards, but does not necessarily reflect the overall quality of care. Core measures alone are not adequate performance measures, but must be considered along with other indicators.

Evaluating Compliance with Internal and External Requirements

CRITICAL PATHWAYS

Critical pathways are multidisciplinary care plans, which outline care steps and expected outcomes, based on the patient's specific diagnosis, procedure, or condition. Critical pathways outline goals in patient care, and the sequence and timing of interventions to achieve those goals. Critical pathways improve and standardize care, and decrease hospital stays. There are two basic types of critical pathways:

- **Guidelines**: No documentation is required to verify that the pathway has been followed. A guideline suggests how to conduct optimal patient care. The guideline is usually a flow sheet, with different If–Then paths to follow, depending on the patient's outcomes.
- **Integrated Care Plan**: An ICP requires dates, signatures, and documentation to show that the steps have been carried out and to indicate specific outcomes.

Write pathways based on best practices. Monitor their effectiveness regularly. Periodically evaluate their outcomes to determine if modifications are needed to reach goals.

Critical pathways are developed by multidisciplinary teams involved in direct patient care. For example, a critical pathway for hip replacements involves a rheumatologist, surgeon, anesthetist, surgical and orthopedic nurses, physiotherapist, occupational therapist, pharmacist, nutritionist, and social worker. The pathway cannot require additional staffing, and must cover the entire scope of an illness in these steps:

- Select a patient group based on data analysis and observations that show:
    - A wide variance in the current treatment approach
    - An organizational priority
    - Increasing patient needs (e.g., more hip replacements because of aging Boomers)
- Create an interdisciplinary pathway development team.
- Review literature. Study best practices. Identify opportunities for quality improvement.
- Identify all categories of care (nutrition, pharmacy, nursing, etc.).
- Discuss findings and reach consensus.
- Identify levels of care and number of days covered by the pathway.
- Pilot test the pathway and redesign steps as required.
- Educate staff.
- Monitor and track variances to improve the pathway.

UTILIZATION REVIEWS

A utilization review (UR) determines whether care was medically necessary at admission, during treatment, and at discharge, and whether it adhered to critical pathways. UR evaluates whether decision-making, care, and length of the hospital stay are appropriate. Third-party payers and insurance companies conduct utilization reviews. Issues considered during UR include the severity of illness based on symptoms, history, and laboratory testing, and the intensity of service, based on diagnostic procedures and treatments. UR may result in legal actions with individual practitioners, such as intervening in care. Appeal processes for those denied coverage for treatments or care must be written and available. Appeals are considered first by an independent reviewer, and if a denial is received, a second review is conducted by independent external reviewers. States have specific regulations dealing with the appeal process.

Utilization Management

Integrating the Outcome of Utilization Management Assessment

The utilization management assessment measures and assesses the use of services, procedures, and facilities in terms of medical necessity and appropriateness. The following trends should be analyzed:

- **Overutilization**: Inappropriate admissions, levels of care, length of stay, or undocumented rationale for resource use (such as frequent, expensive lab tests).
- **Underutilization**: Level of care or resources were inadequate for medical necessity (failure to admit, inadequate lab testing).
- **Misutilization**: Errors were made in treatment, or inefficiencies occurred in scheduling.

Integrating the outcomes of utilization assessment requires intervention strategies, assessment of cost-effectiveness related to quality and risk, consideration of the need to modify the preauthorization process, peer review, and establishment of teams for process improvement. Utilization management (UM) is also an important part of assessing and resolving problems through quality management.

Utilization Management Functions under Quality Management

Utilization management functions that fall under quality management include the following:

- Concurrent assessment of important aspects of patient care.
- Case management to ensure resources are utilized appropriately in patient care.
- Team assessment and review of processes to ensure they are cost-effective and maintain the quality of care.
- Identification of patterns and trends across the organization.
- Practitioner profiling, credentialing, privileging, and re-privileging include coordinated information from all areas of review to provide an objective assessment.

Problems with Utilization Management Hindering Integration of Outcomes

Problems with utilization management that may hinder the integration of outcomes include the following:

- Lack of coordination that interferes with the flow of information
- Medical errors
- Fear of malpractice driving unnecessary testing and utilization of resources
- Lack of cost-knowledge on the part of staff
- Capitation pressure to underutilize
- Lack of adequate community services
- Inadequate data collection

Patient Flow Management

Patient flow management incorporates the outcome of utilization management assessment as it relates to the functions and processes of the organization that impact the quality of patient care. Patient flow management assesses the way the patient moves through the system, from triage and admission to access of services and discharge. Flow includes scheduling concerns and methods of routing patients through services. Departments are interdependent on each other. Only organization-wide utilization management is in the position to evaluate and integrate information and services. For example, admissions depend on discharges, which depend on completed imaging and laboratory studies, which in turn depend on the transmission of orders and patient transport.

Determining where the patient flow processes can be improved and where resources are underutilized, overutilized, or misutilized can drive change that effectively improves patient flow.

CASE MANAGEMENT

Case management is an important tool for integrating the outcome of utilization management assessment into the performance improvement process. Utilization review and management are primarily used to determine cost effectiveness and to contain costs, but that must be balanced by individual patients' needs. The governing board and medical directors of the hospital must determine the criteria for appropriate care, based on the mission and strategic goals of the organization. The case manager screens patients from the time of admission (or before admission in some cases) and assists with discharge planning. In some cases, criteria require that second opinions be rendered before non-emergent surgery. Case managers are involved in all aspects of patient care, across disciplines:

- Assessing the plan of care
- Coordinating treatment and providing continuity
- Providing continuous assessment by evaluating variances to critical pathways
- Completing evaluation and discharge planning
- Performing a post-discharge assessment

MODELS FOR CASE MANAGEMENT

Three models for case management that can be used to integrate the outcome of utilization management assessment into the performance improvement process are:

- **Type of provider care**: Includes self-care by the patient, primary care (patient and primary care physician), episodic care (patient, primary care physician, specialist, and case manager), and brokered care (involves community, government, or private services).
- **Focus of care**: The focus may be on cost containment, common to managed care programs, where service depends on the program's benefits and criteria for medical necessity, and there is little or no direct contact with the patient or family. The focus may also be on coordination of care, which involves direct patient and family contact, and individualized assessment and intervention.
- **Professional discipline**: Case management may be done by nurses, social workers, psychiatrists, or other specific disciplines, depending on the goals of case management.

PROCESS VARIANCE MONITORING

Process variance monitoring is a review that uses critical pathways as a basis for processes involved in medical care. A variance is a deviation from the pathway. The variance may result from a part of the process not being performed or from the process not resulting in anticipated outcomes. Process variance monitoring creates a large amount of data. It is most effective when it is targeted to critical outcomes, where variance negatively impacts patients. Document variances and take corrective steps as necessary. If the purpose is to modify or improve a pathway, variance data should be computerized and aggregated. Process variance monitoring is not used to identify individuals who are at fault, but rather to identify faulty processes.

MEDICAL REVIEW PROCESS

Medical review processes are mandated by regulations and accreditation. **Types** include:

Prospective reviews	Include all those steps taken before an event, such as assessing need before care, checking credentials before hiring, determining ability to pay prior to doing elective procedures, and gaining preauthorization from insurance companies.
Concurrent reviews	Include ongoing assessment while the patient is receiving care, verification of medical necessity for continued treatment, and appropriate use of resources. Concurrent review uses medical records, observations of care, incident reports, and special case studies.
Retrospective reviews	These reviews are conducted after care is completed, and they provide a full picture of the continuum of care and its effectiveness. Medical records and the results of prospective and concurrent reviews are used.
Focused reviews	Include reviews done for specific, predetermined reasons, such as a particular diagnosis, procedure, or process. Criteria for case selection must be clearly outlined.

Develop a flow chart for a **medication usage review**, which lists all steps in the process of medication use and the disciplines involved. This overview is necessary before a more targeted review can be accomplished:

- Process review
- Selecting medications
- Purchase order for supplier
- Receiving
- Storage
- Prescribing
- Transcribing orders
- Ordering from pharmacy
- In-patient unit receiving from pharmacy
- Scanning barcodes
- Preparing and dispensing
- Recording in the computer or patient's chart
- Administration
- Monitoring patient's response to medication

PURPOSE OF A MEDICATION USAGE REVIEW

The physician and pharmacist determine the purpose and scope of a medication review, and methods of data collection. Medication usage reviews are conducted with different parameters, depending on their purpose:

- Determine compliance with accreditation standards
- Evaluate potential cost savings
- Study the correlation of drugs with outcomes to improve patient care
- Evaluate staff education related to best practices
- Detect medication errors, observe error patterns, determine methods to avoid errors, and chart adverse reactions
- Determine if critical pathways have been followed, and to develop further critical pathways or modify existing ones

In addition to medication review, it is important for clinicians to conduct a medication reconciliation, especially after transitions of care, such as when a patient is being discharged from the hospital. Medication reconciliation is an important component of patient safety with the goal of obtaining a complete and accurate list of a patient's current medications. By conducting this thorough assessment, discrepancies can be resolved to ensure patients are receiving accurate treatment.

SCOPE AND DATA COLLECTION

The scope of a medication review directly relates to its purpose. The scope of the review can be:

- Very broad, including quantifying all prescriptions for medications within an organization
- Narrowed to those patients and staff in one area or department
- Focused on individual use of prescribed medications
- Include or exclude outpatient prescriptions
- Include all classes of medications, or focus on one or more, such as antibiotics
- Examine the difference in generic and brand name drug use

Review current tracking methods for adequacy of **data collection**. Paper data collection is extremely time-consuming. If prescriptions and medication dispensing are computerized, then measurements are more accurate and easier to obtain. Consider bar coding, unit dose packaging, automated drug dispensing machines (ADDM) and a computerized recording system that links the Lab, nursing unit, and Pharmacy.

Systematic Approach to Medical Record Reviews

A systematic approach to medical record reviews requires planning and consistency. Surveillance may involve:

- **Targeted medical record review** with reporting forms that include all necessary information in one form, paper or electronic.
- **Standardized questionnaires** designed to obtain quantifiable information, featuring clear, unambiguous, and non-threatening questions. Open-ended questions may be appropriate for some types of information gathering, especially in relation to information that may be embarrassing or that identifies staff errors.
- **Consistent coding** of data collection, with specific codes for units, populations, and individuals to facilitate analysis. Thus, the report of a patient with a cough has the same identification code as the laboratory work for that patient.
- **Electronic surveillance** triggered by threshold data. Reports are directly integrated with the data analysis system.

Depending on the goal of the medical record review, the analysis may be conducted through a chart-based system or a code-based system. **Chart-based systems** are most effective when dealing with a smaller sample size, as this involves an analyst manually reviewing details within the chart to identify requested information. A **code-based system** is most effective when a larger sample size is required for review and encompasses a retrospective review of administrative, standardized data, such as claims information, to identify requested information.

Surveillance Plans

The purpose of a surveillance plan is clearly outlined by the CPHQ and Infection Control Manager. Include the following elements:

- Identify a means to decrease nosocomial infections.
- Evaluate the effectiveness of infection control measures.
- Establish endemic threshold rates and enact control measures to reduce rates. About 5–10% of infections occur in outbreaks, so if the CPHQ analyzes data in a regular and timely manner, it establishes if the disease is endemic or an outbreak.
- Convince staff to cooperate with infection control measures by presenting objective evidence.
- Report infection rates to public health departments, the CDC, and those accreditation agencies that require reports.
- Provide a defense for malpractice suits and decrease liability by accumulating evidence that the facility is proactive in combating infections.
- Compare the facility's infection rates with similar facilities', to focus attention and resources.

Infection Control Surveillance Plan

The steps in an infection control surveillance program are as follows:

13. Establish the parameters and design of the survey by determining what will be surveyed, when, and how, with clear definitions to guide the process.
14. Collect data in a consistent, efficient, and accurate manner, whether manual or automated. Sources include laboratory reports, medical records of targeted patients, interviews, and autopsy reports.
15. Summarize data to make information easily accessible and available for further analysis.

16. Analyze data using statistical measurements appropriate to the data and goals. The frequency of analysis varies but must ensure adequate numbers for the results to be meaningful.
17. Conduct an analytical interpretation of the data, which involves using data to indicate threshold rates, clusters, outbreaks, and adverse events.
18. Utilize results of analytical interpretation to ameliorate the event. For example, if a threshold for infections is exceeded, clearly define procedures for dealing with that event.

ACTIVE AND PASSIVE SURVEILLANCE PLANS

Active surveillance is a program specifically designed for finding nosocomial infections, using trained and certificated staff, such as infection control nurses. Active surveillance is more accurate than passive surveillance because its data is more complete and consistent, since it comes from an established program. However, active surveillance is also expensive because it requires dedicated staff.

Passive surveillance uses observations from medical and laboratory staff to identify and report infections, often requiring the staff to fill out a report and submit it. Passive surveillance often results in misclassification, delays, or failure to report infections because no one is specifically charged with reporting. Staff involved in patient care may not have time to fill out reports.

PATIENT-BASED AND LABORATORY-BASED SURVEILLANCE PLANS

Patient-based surveillance plans revolve around the patient, so the patient must be assessed for signs of infection, risk factors, quality of patient care, and staff compliance with infection control protocols. Patient-based plans are very time and staff intensive, requiring much time on the in-patient units to review charts, assess patients, and interview patients and staff. For large facilities, the cost of effective patient-based plans is prohibitive.

Laboratory-based plans depend on reviews of laboratory findings, usually cultures, to determine if threshold rates are exceeded. Laboratory findings are usually accurate, but the effectiveness of this type of plan depends on completeness of records and whether specimens are correctly collected and sent to the laboratory for analysis. If there are no clear protocols in place to determine when a specimen should be obtained, infections are missed. Lab plans have electronic monitoring systems, saving staff time.

PROSPECTIVE AND RETROSPECTIVE SURVEILLANCE PLANS

Prospective, or concurrent, surveillance follows patients while they are hospitalized and includes the 30-day period after discharge to evaluate for surgical site infections. Because prospective surveillance is ongoing and continually evaluated, it identifies clusters of infection as they occur, ensuring that Infection Control personnel have ongoing working relationships with other staff. When there appears to be an outbreak or cause for concern, analysis can be done fairly quickly.

Retrospective surveillance is conducted after the fact by a review of charts and records, with no patient contact. There is a delay between the time a problem presents and the time it is identified. Retrospective surveillance is less expensive because it is ad hoc.

PRIORITY-DIRECTED AND POST-DISCHARGE SURVEILLANCE

Priority-directed surveillance is also called surveillance by objective. It ranks infection surveillance efforts in order of their importance for meeting particular goals. Serious infections are identified based on morbidity and mortality rates, costs, and the effectiveness of preventive measures based on the data. Therefore, priority-directed surveillance is often directed at surgical site infections and pneumonia. Other infections are not simply ignored, but most resources are expended in focused areas.

Post-discharge surveillance is not standardized, so it misses up to 50% of surgical site infections in patients who have short hospital stays. Patients are contacted directly through mailed questionnaires or by telephone. Sometimes, physicians are contacted for information. Readmission data is evaluated, and in some cases, patients are followed in clinics or office visits. Data is often insufficient because of difficult follow-up.

LIMITATIONS OF TARGETED SURVEILLANCE VS. HOSPITAL-WIDE SURVEILLANCE

The major problem with hospital-wide surveillance is its prohibitive costs in time and money. However, hospital-wide surveillance is necessary to detect all infections and to get a clear idea of the infection control problems at a facility. When the CDC National Nosocomial Infections Surveillance system (NNIS) was in place (1992-2004), it required hospital-wide surveillance, but discontinued this in favor of targeted surveillance because most hospitals could not afford comprehensive surveillance. Infection control still does some hospital-wide surveillance because, for instance, only about 20% of hospital-acquired infections occur in the ICU, the main targeted area. Only about 19% of hospital-acquired infections involve surgical sites. Use an electronic monitoring program that automatically flags suspicious lab results, such as TheraDoc. Create a rotating system for monitoring different units for specified periods of time to gain a more comprehensive picture of infections.

PRE-DESIGNED SURVEILLANCE SOFTWARE

Managing data manually is unwieldy. Use standard spreadsheet software that is packaged with most computers for simple reporting and database functions (e.g., Excel and Access). Multiple variables are more difficult to manage on a spreadsheet, and require extensive customization. Use pre-designed surveillance software packages to save time and expense, and yield more accurate data. Statistical packages, like SAS, SPSS, and MINITAB, have a steep learning curve. The CDC provides the free program Epi Info, which was originally designed for outbreak investigation, but can manage and analyze data. It consists of these programs:

- Nutstat (a nutritional program)
- MakeView (to design data entry screens)
- Enter (to enter data into screens designed with MakeView)
- Epi Map (to link data to maps)
- Data Compare and Epi Report (for various types of statistical analysis)
- Epi Lock for privacy and data compression

POPULATION ASSESSMENT

Assessment of population is a very important component of a surveillance plan because each facility deals with a unique population. Population refers to that segment of patients who will be studied, because studying all patients, especially in large facilities, is impractical. Assessing a population leads to targeted surveillance where particular areas, procedures, or types of patients are surveyed. Assessment means identifying:

- Types of patients for evaluation, including medical and surgical, and frequent diagnoses
- Commonly performed procedures and treatments, especially those that are invasive
- Liability issues in relation to those patients that affect liability and costs
- Community health issues, such as outbreaks, to target populations

- Risk factors for infection as part of needs assessment
- Facility resources and support because staff assistance is critical

JOINT COMMISSION'S ROLE IN THE DEVELOPMENT OF INFECTION CONTROL PROGRAMS

The Joint Commission accredits most healthcare facilities in the United States. It established a requirement in 1969 that hospitals have both committees for infection control and isolation facilities in response to a growing concern about hospital-acquired infections. The Joint Commission plans to "reduce the risk of health care-associated infections" to both patients and health care workers. The Joint Commission lists extensive standards for surveillance, prevention, and control of infection with which healthcare facilities must comply. These guidelines and an organized infection control program are explicit accreditation requirements. Many healthcare facilities incorporate Joint Commission wording regarding infections into their infection control mission statement. Hospitals are given an accreditation report that is publicly listed, showing their compliance with goals established by the Joint Commission. Joint Commission International accredits hospitals throughout the world.

NOSOCOMIAL INFECTIONS

Nosocomial infection is defined by the National Healthcare Safety Network (NHSN) as a hospital-acquired infection, either localized or systemic, caused by a pathogen or toxin that was not present (or incubating) in the patient at the time he or she entered the hospital. Some infections are obvious within the first 24–48 hours, but other infections may not be obvious until after discharge from the hospital because incubation times and resistance vary. An infection that occurs within 30 days after discharge, but is hospital-acquired, is considered nosocomial. Nosocomial infections are identified from analysis of laboratory results and clinical signs and symptoms. A diagnosis of infection by an attending physician or surgeon is also considered acceptable identification. Placentally-transferred infections are not considered nosocomial, but perinatal infections are, even if acquired from the mother during delivery. Colonization that is not causing an inflammatory response or evidence of infection is not considered nosocomial for reporting purposes.

DETERMINING THE INCIDENCE OF NOSOCOMIAL INFECTIONS

The incidence of nosocomial infections during a specific time period is the number of new infections (numerator) in a population at risk (denominator) during the same time period. The incidence rate is the number of events (numerator) divided by the number of the population at risk (denominator), often expressed as the number of infections per 100 patients. Incidence may also be used to calculate incidence density, which is the rate at which disease occurs in relation to the size of the population without disease. Incidence density uses the number of infections (numerator) in relation to units of time (denominator), such as the number of infections that occur in 1,000 patient days. Incidence may also be used to calculate attack rate, expressed as a percentage of a population at risk (denominator data) over a given time period.

CDC DEFINITIONS FOR NOSOCOMIAL INFECTIONS

In 1988, the Centers for Disease Control established the CDC Definitions for Nosocomial Infections to standardize reporting and obtain meaningful data for a national database. Definitions include:

- **Infection site**: For example, a urinary tract infection is coded as UTI and a surgical site infection is coded as SSI.
- **Code**: The site of infection is further coded according to the sub-type: SUTI, symptomatic urinary tract infection; ASB, asymptomatic bacteriuria; and OUTI, other infections of the urinary tract.

The definition of the infection outlines the criteria for inclusion into a coded category. For example, UTI-SUTI (urinary tract infection–symptomatic urinary tract infection) includes 3 different criteria. Criterion 2 is defined as:

- Patient has at least 1 of the following signs or symptoms with no other recognized cause: Fever (>38 °C), urgency, frequency, dysuria, costovertebral tenderness, or suprapubic tenderness.

USING STANDARDIZED DEFINITIONS

For internal or external comparison data to be valid there must be **consistency in definitions** as to what comprises a nosocomial infection, including onset, symptoms, and laboratory findings. Clear definitions must be in place for events, indicators, and outcomes.

- **Events** are usually defined according to the CDC definitions for nosocomial infections, but if the institution has other definitions they must be used consistently and cannot then be compared to events using other definitions.
- **Indicators** are a measure of quality because they represent numerator data (the number of events that are being targeted, such as specific types of infections, defined as narrowly as possible). The denominator data is the population at risk for the indicator event.
- **Outcomes** are measurements of indicators, such as the number of infections per a specified denominator, such as 100 patient days, or 1,000 device days. Outcomes should provide feedback.

NATIONAL NOSOCOMIAL INFECTIONS SURVEILLANCE (NNIS)

In 1970, the National Centers for Infectious Diseases of the US Centers for Disease Control and Prevention (CDC) established the National Nosocomial Infections Surveillance (NNIS) system. The purposes were to encourage hospitals to report and track nosocomial infections, to use standardized methods to collect and analyze data, and to create a national database. About 300 hospitals, whose identity remained confidential, reported data using "surveillance components" and protocols that had been standardized and used CDC definitions. Surveillance components included:

- Adult and pediatric Intensive Care Units (ICUs)
- High-risk nurseries (HRN)
- Surgical patients
- Antimicrobial use and resistance

All ICU and HRN patients were surveyed, but hospitals chose from a list of surgical procedures those that they wanted to monitor for surgical patients, as the numbers of procedures done at different hospitals vary widely. Infection statistics were compiled and reported every 3 years. In 2004 this system was absorbed into the National Healthcare Safety Network (NHSN), now responsible for conducting and generating surveillance reports on nosocomial infections.

Customers

A **customer**, in the general sense of the term, is a receiver. When it comes to health care quality assurances, there are various categories of customers that must be considered:

- **Internal customers** are those directly involved in product or healthcare delivery, such as the board of directors, administrators, clerical staff, nurses, medical support staff, physicians, human resources personnel, plant managers, pharmacists, and volunteer staff. Internal customers need others in the work environment to provide some type of product or service in order for them to function, and they, in turn, provide a product or service to others, so each internal customer is also a supplier.
  - Vertical customer/supplier relationships, such as between administration and nursing staff, are sometimes more obvious than the equally important horizontal relationships, such as between floor nurses, which involve cooperative measures to ensure that quality care is provided. Identify these types of customer/supplier relationships in the strategic plan to help increase internal awareness and improve methods of meeting the various customers' needs.
- **External customers** are critical to an organization because these customers are those that receive products or services supplied by the organization's workers. External customers include patients and their families, private physicians, vendors, insurance companies, government regulatory agencies, lawyers, and others in the community.
  - As with internal customers, each external customer is both a receiver of products or services and a supplier. For example, a regulatory agency provides regulations and guidelines as a supplier, and then receives reports in return as a customer. This symbiotic relationship must be clearly understood by the CPHQ, because the external customer-supplier relationship is one over which the organization often has less direct control, so identification of the customers' needs through surveys, interviews, focus groups, research, and brainstorming can help to clarify and improve these relationships.

Assessing Customer Needs
Teams

Teams can assess customer needs as both providers and customers, so their perspective is different than that of focus groups. Teams should be interdisciplinary. Members should represent all the different steps in a process, in order to better understand the needs of the customers. Because team members are actively involved in the process and share objectives, even though their individual responsibilities differ, they are concerned for the customers and can generate ideas about change and reach consensus from a solid knowledge base. Teams meet and discuss issues related to customer needs, identifying customers, sharing perspectives, and generating lists of recommendations for process improvement. A team leader is responsible for keeping members focused on task, and ensures that all members participate, rather than one or two dominating the meetings. The team leader is also responsible for summarizing and reporting findings related to assessment.

Surveys

Surveys are valuable tools to assess both customer needs and improvement progress. Take care with the survey design, because it must have validity. Before beginning, decide on the following variables:

- **Target group**: Who will receive the survey? Do you need an entire population of customers (e.g., all discharge patients), or only a percentage (e.g., 30% of discharges from the emergency department), or some other sampling? Identifying the target group can be complex.
- **Type of survey**: There are different investments of time and money for paper, telephone, and internet surveys, so check the budget.
- **Type of questions**: Questions with a yes/no decision are usually easier to quantify than open-ended questions or scales, although scales are frequently used to assess the degree of satisfaction.
- **Format**: Do font size, color, and general layout comply with the Americans with Disabilities Act (ADA)?
- **Follow-up**: Survey completion rates are often low. Think up incentives for people to complete surveys. Prepare reminder letters if receiving a low response.

Peer Review

Joint Commission's Focus on Peer Review

Peer review is an examination of one practitioner by a like practitioner who has similar training, experience, and expertise. If the pool of practitioners is too small within an organization, arrange an external peer review. Peer review is often triggered by root cause analysis that indicates the need to focus on an individual, sometimes related to utilization review. A peer review is effective when it is defensible, balanced, and consistent. The Joint Commission focuses on the process of peer review in both design and function:

The **design** includes:

- A definition of a peer
- The method for selecting the peer review panel
- Triggering events
- Timeframes
- An outline of how the person being reviewed participates
- Decisions based on solid reason and literature review

The **function** is:

- Consistently applied to all individuals
- Balanced and fair
- Adherent to timelines
- Ongoing
- Valuable to the organization
- Defensible

Participation in Peer Review

Peer review is an intensive process in which an individual practitioner is reviewed by like practitioners. Peer review can examine the practitioner's work with an individual patient or a group of patients, and often relates to data found as part of root cause analysis, infection control, or other surveillance measures. A ranking system indicates **compliance** with standards:

- Care is based on standards and is typical of that provided by like practitioners.
- Variance in care occurs, but outcomes are satisfactory.
- Care is inconsistent with that provided by like practitioners.
- Variance resulted in negative outcomes.
- In some cases, this ranking system is replaced with a series of questions, with affirmative answers indicating cause for concern.

Impact of the Healthcare Quality Improvement Act (HCQIA) on Peer Review

Congress passed the **HCQIA of 1986** to ensure the quality of medical care by reviews, and to discipline physicians providing poor quality care or who engage in unprofessional conduct. HCQIA confers limited immunity on those engaged in the peer review process if they follow the procedural provisions of the Act to ensure fairness. HCQIA created the **National Practitioner Data Bank**, so that incompetent individuals must be reported, preventing them from simply moving practice to another state, and requiring organizations to request information about physicians applying for work. Prior to the passage of HCQIA, physicians involved in peer review were subject to antitrust lawsuits for using the process to decrease competition. Practitioners are evaluated by **peer review** when:

- They apply for membership or reappointment.
- Root cause analysis or complaints about an individual physician set off a trigger.

The potential for abuse exists in peer review, so ensure that the organization rigorously follows federal and state regulations.

Practitioner Profiling

Practitioner profiling provides practitioner-specific data and an information summary as part of reappraisal for recredentialing or re-privileging. Ideally, this is an ongoing process, or is performed every 1-2 years, as required for credentialing. Profiling documents both areas of concern and positive outcomes, must remain confidential, and is released only according to the bylaws of the organization and for peer review. Reviews must be signed by appropriate management/supervisory staff, such as medical directors. Profiles should include the following information:

- Clinical monitoring, including mortality rates and peer-reviewed events with negative ratings
- Practices placing patients at risk, including operative procedures, medications, and blood product administration
- Healthcare-related infection rates
- Utilization management findings, including readmissions and average length of stay (ALOS)
- Patient safety findings related to root cause analysis
- Findings of risk management and medical record reviews

EMPLOYEE PERFORMANCE APPRAISAL SYSTEM

Performance appraisal is a supervisory function used to confirm hiring, promote, train, or reward staff. It should be performed when the employee's probationary period ends and on an annual basis thereafter. Supervisors who perform the appraisal should use objective data and standards, and should know and have observed the employee who is being appraised. Review the employee's job description first, which includes expectations and goals related to performance. Indicate in the written appraisal if the employee complies with performance expectations. Determine the role the employee has in processes and incorporate findings from performance improvement measures in the evaluation. The appraisal form may include a rating scale, checklist, productivity studies, and narrative. Discuss the appraisal with the employee, so he or she has an opportunity to respond. The employee must establish new goals, based on findings from performance improvement measures and related to strategic plans of the organization.

INCORPORATING FINDINGS FROM PERFORMANCE IMPROVEMENT

Findings from performance improvement are increasingly part of credentialing, appointments, and privileging delineation, as clinical guidelines and accountability have become accepted medical practice. Consider how the individual practitioner adheres to standards. Clinical privileges are delineated based on criteria established by the organization, and are specific to the practitioner's area of expertise. Privilege control sheets outline the level of competency necessary for each privilege granted. Competency levels are based on best practices and performance improvement data. Privileges are granted for a specific period of time, and not for the lifetime of the practitioner. The Joint Commission sets continuing education requirements for accreditation and demands documented completion of continuing education courses for credentialing.

PATHOLOGY REVIEWS

Pathology services are of critical importance to the healthcare organization because the majority of healthcare decisions for most patients are based on clinical pathology. Review topics of particular concern to pathology include:

- **Technology**: Outline the degree and type of automated testing, computerized reporting, and linkage to all departments within the organization.
- **Patient safety**: Describe monitoring, supervision, adequate staffing, consistent practices to ensure quality, and use of unique patient identifier numbers to prevent mistakes in matching samples with patients' records.
- **Productivity**: Cover the time from ordering to delivery of laboratory reports, hours of operation, phlebotomy and sample collection, laboratory layout, workflow efficiency, satellite bleeding stations for sample collection, reference laboratories, and transport methods for samples.

RADIOLOGY REVIEWS

Radiology may also be called Medical Imaging if it includes not only x-rays, but also CT, MRI, fluoroscopy, ultrasound, and Nuclear Medicine. Review topics of particular concern to Radiology include:

- **Scope**: The variety of services offered and whether they are sufficient for the population and the needs of the organization, including physicians.
- **Point-of-care**: Satellite departments and portable imaging equipment that is taken to the patient's bedside facilitate access better than a central Radiology department.
- **Accuracy**: Experienced radiologists must be available to identify abnormal findings and stage tumors.

- **Productivity**: Cover the time from the order to generation of a report, and list the number of patients accommodated, hours of operation and staffing, cost-effectiveness, and patient satisfaction with services.
- **Safety measures**: Describe how staff, patients, and others are protected from excess radiation, injury, and pain.

PHARMACY REVIEWS

Pharmacy reviews must consider the broader context of medication management throughout the organization, rather than just the processes within the pharmacy. Topics for review include:

- Use of evidence-based practices in building the formulary
- Procedures and safeguards for administration of medications, including identification of drugs through labeling, bar-coding, or other methods, and matching to appropriate patients
- Compliance with regulations and accreditation standards
- Error rates in dispensing and administration of drugs
- Education and training provided to staff about new medications/treatments
- Procedures for ensuring medication safety and proper storage
- Policies for investigational or off-label medications
- Point-of-care in providing prescribed medications
- Efficiency and time from order to medication delivery

NURSING REVIEWS

Nursing reviews evaluate registered nurses and licensed practical nurses in relation to accreditation standards, which vary slightly from one state to another. Nurses must focus on providing good quality care. Topics for review include:

- Ethical behavior and respect for patients' rights
- Infection control methods
- Effective collaboration with physicians and other healthcare providers
- Clear, legal, informative, and timely medical record documentation
- Adherence to nursing standards, and competency
- Data collection and measurements
- Staff-patient ratios in different departments
- Orientation, training, continuing education, nursing licensure and certification
- Safety, including prevention of patient falls, injury, and ulcers, and proper administration of medications
- Incident reports
- Patient assessments and nursing diagnoses
- Pain management

GOVERNMENT REGULATION DEALING WITH COMPLAINTS, GRIEVANCES, AND APPEALS

Healthcare organizations that participate in federal programs, such as Medicare or Medicaid, must have procedures in place for patient complaints, grievances, and appeals as a condition of participation. Under this regulation, the governing board assigns a team to receive all complaints, rather than an individual. Patients must be notified of their right to file complaints, grievances, and appeals. Additional state regulations vary.

- **Complaint**: A specific oral or written report of lack of satisfaction with the quality of care or processes of care by a patient, guardian, or non-union staff member; a written complaint is the first step in a civil or criminal court proceeding.
- **Grievance**: If a complaint is not resolved, it progresses to a grievance, which is a formal written complaint about contract violation, quality of care, or financial issues by a union member.
- **Appeal**: When a complaint or grievance is found invalid by an organization, the complainant or griever asks for an impartial review of the decision from a third party.

COMPLAINT ANALYSIS

A process for filing complaints, grievances, and appeals must be in place in healthcare organizations. Performing and/or coordinating complaint analysis includes investigation and response. These are the CPHQ's related duties:

- Receive formal complaints by the designated process, usually in writing.
- Categorize complaints by type of complaint and department or area of concern.
- Establish a timeframe for complaint resolution.
- Assign the complaint to the appropriate department.
- Investigate quality care issues, including a medical record review, interviews with those involved in the process, and onsite observations.
- Review any bylaws or regulations that may impact decisions.
- Generate reports and respond to the complaint.
- Maintain the confidentiality of files.
- Communicate with upper management, leadership, and risk management.
- Provide guidance for performance improvement based on findings.
- Prepare remedial training materials and present training classes.

PATIENT/CUSTOMER SATISFACTION

Patient/customer satisfaction is usually measured with surveys given to patients on discharge from an institution or on completion of treatment. One problem with analyzing surveys is that establishing benchmarks is difficult because so many different survey and data collection methods are used that comparison data may be meaningless. Internal benchmarking is more effective, but the sample rate for surveys may not be sufficient to provide validity. As patients become more knowledgeable and their demand for accountability increases, patient satisfaction is being used as a guide for performance improvement, although patient perceptions of clinical care do not always correlate with outcomes. Survey results provide feedback that makes healthcare providers more aware of customer expectations. Currently, surveys are most often used to evaluate **service** elements of care, rather than clinical elements. Analysis includes:

- Determining the patient/customer's degree of trust
- Determining the degree of satisfaction with care/treatment
- Identifying unmet needs
- Identifying patient/customer priorities

COMMUNICATION IN INCIDENT INVESTIGATION

Communication is a critical issue in incident investigation because accurate information must be collected and disseminated in a timely manner:

- Notify the investigation team members of the incident immediately, so they can begin to assist with the investigation, according to their role in the team.
- Notify all physicians, managers, administrators, and staff who are involved. Ask them to assist by reporting new incidents. Update them frequently.
- Contact the laboratory very early in the investigation. Alert the lab staff to save specimens as necessary for further testing. Laboratory staff can provide information about laboratory procedures that are germane to the incident.
- If necessary, notify and involve ancillary staff, such as housekeepers or food workers.
- Notify city, county, state, or federal officials, as the type of incident requires.

COMMUNICATING FINDINGS

All members of an organization should be provided access to **performance improvement information** with which they are involved. Management must ensure that confidentiality is maintained, so remove patient identifiers and practitioners' names from the data. Peer review activities must follow state regulations. Store peer review records separately from those disseminated. Provide reports to upper management and the governing board at quarterly meetings. Ask managers to disseminate reports through staff meetings. Also provide an annual summary report that tracks progress. Give teams, departments, and leaders feedback on performance measures. Use newsletters, email, or the intranet to post performance information. Include contact information for those who wish to comment or ask questions, which encourages organization-wide participation. Ask the IT department how to ensure that sensitive information does not leave the organization by electronic means.

CHANGES IN POLICIES, PROCEDURES, AND WORKING STANDARDS

Changes in policies, procedures, or working standards are common, and the CPHQ is responsible for effectively educating the staff about changes related to processes in a timely manner:

- **Policies** are usually changed after a period of discussion and review by administration and staff. Make all staff aware that a policy change is under discussion. Disseminate preliminary information to staff regarding the issue during meetings or through printed notices.
- **Procedures** are connected to policy changes and are made to increase efficiency or improve patient safety, often as the result of surveillance and data about outcomes. Advertise procedural changes with posters, explain them in workshops with demonstrations, and give handouts to reinforce training.
- **Working standards** are changed in accordance with regulatory or accrediting requirements. Cover working standards extensively with discussions, workshops, and handouts so staff clearly understands the implications of non-compliance.

COMPILING AND WRITING PERFORMANCE IMPROVEMENT REPORTS

Establish formal procedures for compiling and writing performance improvement reports for each department or area with reporting responsibilities. Include the timeline for reports (usually monthly or quarterly). Summarize monthly reports in quarterly master reports. Written reports should include:

- Applicable organization-wide data
- Data relevant to the reporting entity

- Department-specific data for comparisons (e.g., diagnoses, demographics, morbidity, infection rates, stay lengths, external reviews, unplanned events, complaints, and incident reports)

Update and compile data at least monthly, even if reports are given only quarterly, so that sentinel events or outcome changes are noted and early interventions conducted. Present all reports with graphics to demonstrate comparisons. Write narratives to describe procedures. Discuss the impact of the data. Tie data to the strategic plan and goals of the organization, so that the report clearly outlines what the purpose of the data is in relation to the master plan.

TEAM REPORTS

Team reports are central to performance improvement. Written documentation must include the following:

- **Team charters** outline essential information about each team (operating dates, members, advisors, purpose, goals, measures, and expected outcomes). The degree of detail varies, but each charter must contain all pertinent information, such as financial and resource needs, and financial impact on the organization.
- **Quarterly and annual reports** for each performance improvement project. Begin with a statement of the desired outcomes. List process tools. Provide information about the status of the project, including data sources, and analysis methods and results.
- **Summary reports** presented in an accessible manner (electronically, in poster form, or on a storyboard). Clarify the problem with a description of actions, outcomes, and evaluation. Use charts, dashboards, or graphs whenever possible, to provide a graphic explanation.

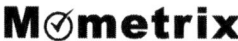

Maintaining Confidentiality

CONFIDENTIALITY

Maintaining confidentiality of performance improvement activities, records, and reports is mandated by state and federal regulations:

- The **Health Insurance Portability and Accountability Act (HIPAA)** protects patients' right to privacy and confidentiality of patient records. An organization can use patients' records for internal quality performance activities, such as monitoring for infections, without obtaining a specific, written authorization signed by the patient or guardian. The governing board, healthcare personnel involved in direct patient care, supervisory staff, and quality teams are allowed access to patients' medical information. When patient information is part of records or reports that will be shared externally, remove the identifying patient information.
- The **Health Care Quality Improvement Act (HCQIA)** provides privacy protection for healthcare organizations and personnel engaged in formal peer review procedures, such as accreditation and performance improvement activities, because confidentiality and immunity further the quality of healthcare. Exclude identifying information from reports and records. Certain conditions apply, and personnel are not exempted from lawsuits for criminal actions.

> **Review Video: HIPAA**
> Visit mometrix.com/academy and enter code: 412009

REQUIRED CONFIDENTIALITY AGREEMENTS AND CONFLICT OF INTEREST STATEMENTS

The CPHQ must inform staff about regulations and correct reporting methods to maintain the confidentiality of performance improvement activities and records. When staff members understand confidentiality issues, it lessens some of their concerns about their performance reviews. Most organizations require personnel who review medical records or participate in performance improvement activities to sign **confidentiality agreements,** which outline privacy issues and increase awareness of confidentiality concerns. Each healthcare organization must have a **conflict-of-interest policy** in place to ensure that reviewers are not primary caregivers and do not have an economic or personal interest in a case under review. Limit access to protected health information to those who need the information to complete their duties related to direct care, or to performance improvement review activities.

MAINTAINING THE CONFIDENTIALITY OF PERFORMANCE-RELATED DATA

Performance improvement teams generate **reports** on a regular basis, which can be monthly, quarterly, or annually, depending on the size of the institution, the population numbers, or device days. Statistics must include adequate **denominator data** for meaningful analysis, and this can require a longer period of time. Specific data about individual patients and healthcare workers are protected by privacy laws (e.g., HIPAA), so do not disseminate information about individuals unless their anonymity is assured. Provide **confidential reports** to individual physicians about their own effectiveness rates. When presenting comparison rates, do not identify the other physicians. Present reports to the administration, teams, and staff in the areas surveyed. Thus, if a quality study involved an ICU, make the ICU staff and physicians aware of the study results, so they can evaluate the effectiveness of their procedures or institute preventive methods.

Regulatory and Accreditation

Accreditation, Certification, and Recognition Options

Accreditation and regulatory recommendations should always be considered minimal, rather than optimal, standards for an organization. View the surveyors' recommendations from the perspective that the institution has failed to meet minimum standards. Use positive reports as part of rewards and positive performance appraisals. Recommendations should trigger these responses to integrate the recommendations into the organization:

- Administrative commitment to utilize resources to meet and exceed recommendations
- Organization-wide education of standards and compliance issues
- Root cause analysis to determine areas of improvement
- Utilization of analysis as part of peer review and/or performance appraisal
- Planning and development of action plans for improvement
- Implementation of action plans
- Ongoing assessment and modification of plans as needed to achieve target outcomes
- Evaluation of action plans in a report to the governing board

ACCREDITATION

ACCREDITATION PROCESSES

Accreditation is an authorization or approval an organization receives once achieving specific standards related to patient care and quality. Accreditation is a primary requirement for most healthcare organizations, because it establishes a commitment to standards based on evaluation. General accreditation is done by one or several of the following:

- The **Joint Commission** accredits more than 22,000 healthcare programs, both nationally and internationally. It is the primary accrediting agency in the United States, so accreditation by the Joint Commission indicates a commitment to improving care and provides information about compliance with core measures.
- The **Healthcare Facilities Accreditation Program of the American Osteopathic Association** also accredits many healthcare programs, including acute care, ambulatory care, rehabilitation centers and substance abuse centers, behavioral care centers, and critical access hospitals. It provides guidelines for patient safety initiatives, and reports common deficiencies.
- **The National Committee for Quality Assurance (NCQA)** offers accreditation to health plans and other organizations in areas such as case management, long-term support services, population health management and utilization management.
- The **Utilization Review Accreditation Commission (URAC)** accredits healthcare delivery systems based on improving health care activities within their organizations. Areas of accreditation include pharmacy, patient care management, administrative management, digital health and telehealth, health plan, and mental health and substance use disorder parity.
- The **Healthcare Facilities Accreditation Program** offers a range of accreditation for different types of healthcare organizations. These include accreditation for acute care hospitals, ambulatory surgery centers, behavioral/mental health, clinical laboratory, critical access hospitals, and office-based surgery.

A healthcare organization may also seek accreditation by agencies with a narrower focus to demonstrate excellence in a particular area, such as the Intersocietal Commission for the Accreditation of Echocardiography Laboratories (ICAEL). Leadership must determine what type of accreditation is most appropriate, based on the programs they offer and their commitment to improvement.

The distinction between accreditation and certification is important for healthcare quality professionals to understand. Certification is a voluntary process, providing a guarantee that certain requirements or standards are met. Accreditation is considered a higher level of achievement, allowing organizations to demonstrate a level of recognition for conforming to standards.

OBTAINING ACCREDITATION

As the first step to obtaining accreditation, the institution performs a **self-assessment** to ensure it complies with standards related to patient care, safety issues, and performance-based core measures (comparative measurements).

Surveyors then perform a peer review to assess compliance. They scrutinize the following:

- Documents (e.g., policies & procedures manuals)
- Medical records
- Standards implementation measures
- Integration of performance measurement data
- Service and support systems
- On-site evaluation activities (inspection, observation, and staff interviews)

The surveyors release their final **report**, which may:

- Renew accreditation
- Make a conditional accreditation (CA) or preliminary denial of accreditation (PDA) if there are infractions
- Make a denial of accreditation (DA) if circumstances pose a threat to staff, the public, or patients

The institution may appeal for **reconsideration** of the surveyors' adverse decision within 60 days. Surveyors conduct a second visit for CA institutions to ensure that infractions are corrected. If the appeal is denied, the institution can request a formal hearing by the FDA to demonstrate its compliance through documentation or interviews.

CPHQ'S ROLE IN ACCREDITATION AND LICENSURE

To obtain accreditation and licensure, a facility must meet standards set by all its regulatory agencies. For example, the Joint Commission evaluates infection control, visiting rules, patient rights, background checks, educational programs, staffing levels, medical records, and ventilation for accreditation. The guidelines by which hospitals are evaluated are very specific, such as the exact minutes after admission for pneumonia that a patient receives an antibiotic, with scores according to the elapsed time. The CPHQ reviews, understands, communicates, and establishes guidelines for all accreditation requirements to ensure all staff and departments are aware of the requirements and document compliance. The accreditation surveyor uses tracer methodology to evaluate the processes that are in place, so complete extensive staff training at all levels regarding processes. Use tracer methodology as part of the general assessment, so staff can practice gathering the type of information they need to supply to the accreditation surveyors.

Appropriate Accreditation, Certification, and Recognition Options

Accreditation Association for Ambulatory Health Care (AAAHC)

The Accreditation Association for Ambulatory Health Care (AAAHC) provides voluntary accreditation for a wide range of ambulatory care providers, including ambulatory surgery centers, dental group practices, diagnostic imaging centers, HMOs, podiatry practices, and women's health centers. AAAHC provides accreditation to the organization itself but also provides specialty-focused certification, such as orthopedic certification. For accreditation, the organization must undergo self-evaluation, peer review, ongoing education, and an on-site survey by AAAHC at least every 3 years.

Commission on Accreditation of Rehabilitation Facilities (CARF)

The Commission on Accreditation of Rehabilitation Facilities (CARF) provides voluntary accreditation to health and human service organizations, such as aging services, behavioral health, medical rehabilitation, opioid treatment programs, and child and youth services. Accreditation requires consultation with a CARF resource specialist for assistance with preparation, self-evaluation, application, payment of a fee, and a survey by CARF surveyors. Accreditation may be provisional or for one to three years. To receive accreditation, the organization must conform to internationally accepted standards.

DNV

DNV is an accreditation organization based in Norway that accredits hospitals, critical access hospitals, and ancillary services, such as home health, hospice, DMEPOS, pharmacy, and private duty. DNV also provides a number of certificates, including infection prevention, stroke care certification, sterile processing certification, orthopedic center of excellence, foot and ankle surgery program certification, spine surgery program certification, cardiac center of excellence, chest pain program certification, extracorporeal program certification, heart failure program certification, VAD facility credentialing, and palliative care program certification. DNV utilizes the National Integrated Accreditation for Healthcare (NIAHO) requirements and integrates CMS Conditions of Participation—qualifications that organizations are required to meet to participate in Medicare, Medicaid, etc., and to achieve deemed status—with the ISO 9001 Quality Management program. Surveys are conducted annually.

International Organization for Standardization (ISO)

The International Organization for Standardization (ISO) publishes international standards. ISO 9000 includes standards for quality management and promotes a process approach utilizing the PDCA cycle and risk-based thinking. Standards are purchased for use by an organization. **ISO 9001:2015** establishes necessary criteria for quality management with a focus on seven quality management principles:

- Customer focus
- Leadership
- Engagement of people
- Process approach
- Improvement
- Evidence-based decision making
- Relationship management

Licensure

While accreditation processes are voluntary, licensure is mandatory, usually through the State Department of Health Services. Hospitals and laboratories must comply with state and federal laws and regulations in order to be licensed. Managed care organizations are usually licensed by other state departments, such as the Department of Insurance. There are a number of different types of licenses, and these vary slightly from one state to another:

- Acute medical and psychiatric hospitals
- Ambulatory surgical centers
- Skilled nursing facilities and sub-acute care centers
- Long-term care facilities
- Home health care agencies
- Hospice agencies
- Assisted living programs
- Residential programs for the behaviorally, mentally, and developmentally disabled

Organizations that use beds or staffing in non-compliant ways risk losing their licenses. Licenses specify the number of patient beds, the types of patients, and staffing provisions, which vary from state to state.

CREDENTIALING AND PRIVILEGING PROCESSES

Credentialing is a background check to verify a job candidate's diplomas, registrations, licenses, references, insurance, and other factors that determine his or her fitness to provide patient care, in accordance with the organization's bylaws. Credentialing covers three critical areas: practitioners, privilege, and place.

Privileging follows the credentialing process and grants the individual authority to practice within the organization. There are five types of privileging:

- **Provisional** privileges are granted during the initial probationary period. It is during this time period that clinical skills and qualifications are assessed.
- **Active** privileges are for staff providing direct care as a primary job function.
- **Consulting** privileges are for staff providing medical services on a periodic or episodic basis.
- **Temporary** privileges are granted for a short period of time in exceptional circumstances.
- **Emergency** privileges are for unique circumstances, such as situations that would place a patient at risk of harm if action was not taken.

Many organizations use internet services to verify credentials (e.g., Kroll Background America and IntelliSoft Group). The credentials committee determines what credentials are necessary for different positions, based on the following:

- Professional standards, such as those of the American Nurses Association
- Licensure
- Regulatory guidelines, such as state requirements
- Accreditation guidelines

Other considerations include best practices, economic considerations, malpractice insurance coverage, disciplinary actions, and organizational needs. Ensure a policy is in place for privileging temporary staff for special circumstances or for emergencies that follows the state's regulations.

CORE CRITERIA

There are many considerations for credentialing and privileging, some of which are internal organizational considerations that do not involve the quality of the applicant. However, four **primary core criteria** focus only on the applicant:

- **Licensure** must be current through the appropriate state board, such as the state board of nursing.
- **Education** is training and experience appropriate for the credential, and can be vocational, technical, professional, residencies, internships, fellowships, doctoral and postdoctoral programs, and board and clinical certifications.
- **Competence** is determined by evaluations and recommendations from peers regarding clinical competency, judgment, and how the candidate applies knowledge.
- **Performance ability**: The candidate must have demonstrated the ability to perform the duties to which the credentialing/privileging applies.

GENERAL COMPETENCIES ADAPTED BY THE JOINT COMMISSION FOR CREDENTIALING AND PRIVILEGING

General competencies for practitioners in healthcare organizations have been adapted by the Joint Commission and apply to all healthcare settings. Competencies necessary for practice under the Focused Practitioner Professional Evaluation (FPPE) include:

- **Patient care**: Patient care provided must be compassionate, appropriate, effective, and must promote health, treat disease, and provide end-of-life support.
- **Medical/clinical knowledge**: The applicant demonstrates knowledge of current and evolving medical, social, and clinical sciences, is able to apply this to patient care, and can use this knowledge to educate others.
- **Practice-based learning and improvement**: Practice-based learning skills, based on scientific methods, should be used to improve patient care.
- **Interpersonal and communication skills**: The applicant uses interpersonal and communication skills to establish and maintain professional relationships with others.
- **Professionalism**: The applicant demonstrates commitment to professional development, ethical practice, and sensitivity to diversity.
- **Systems-based practice**: The applicant understands all aspects of a system and can use knowledge to improve health care.

FPPE should be completed when new privileges are granted and within a time period determined by leadership. Ongoing Professional Practice Evaluation (OPPE) should be completed with a frequency determined by leadership that does not exceed every 12 months.

EXTERNAL RECOGNITION

BALDRIGE AWARD CRITERIA FOR PROCESS MANAGEMENT

The Malcolm Baldrige National Quality Award criteria for process management are models used to facilitate process selection. This award system, based on the Baldrige Performance Excellence Framework, has established standards of review for successful performance regarding quality and performance improvement. Baldrige reviews process management related to work systems design, work process management and improvement, core competencies, disaster preparedness, customers' needs and expectations, decision-making, performance measures, and innovations. Baldrige also reviews the organization's performance and improvement in the following areas:

- Key healthcare outcomes, including comparative data
- Current levels and trends in patient and other customer satisfaction
- Financial performance and market share
- Process effectiveness outcomes
- Leadership outcomes related to carrying out strategic plans, compliance with accreditation and regulatory bodies, and contributions to the community

APPLYING FOR A MALCOLM BALDRIGE NATIONAL QUALITY AWARD

The program reviews applicants based on core values and concepts, systematic processes, and performance results.

Core Values and Concepts	Systematic Processes	Performance Results
Systems perspective Visionary leadership Customer-focused excellence Valuing people Agility and resilience Organizational learning Focus on success and innovation Management by fact Societal contributions Ethics and transparency Delivering value and results	Leadership Operations Workforce Customers Measurement, analysis, and knowledge management Strategy	Leadership and governance results Product and process results Workforce results Customer results Financial, market, and strategy results

Organizations that are in the process of change for performance improvement may apply for the award. Even if an organization does not win, it will benefit from the comprehensive evaluation and objective external review of data that the examiners provide. Reviewers award points. Almost half of 1,000 points pertain to outcomes, so the organization focuses on the most important performance measures. The application process includes an extensive self-assessment that provides a valuable tool for the organization. Essentially, the Baldrige award process serves as an inexpensive consulting service. To fully benefit from the review, an organization must have already begun the work of performance improvement, with action plans developed and activities in place.

ANCC MAGNET STATUS

The **American Nurses' Credentialing Center (ANCC) Magnet Status Award** is given to healthcare organizations based on their quality of nursing care. An extensive self-assessment is required as part of the application process, which provides valuable information about nursing within the organization. The actual review provides feedback to facilitate change. However, many criteria must be met before an organization is eligible for a Magnet award.

There are 5 components to the Magnet program that must be addressed to demonstrate expertise and knowledge:

- **Transformational leadership** focuses on agility and how leaders can best transform their organizations to be prepared for unprecedented demands in the future.
- **Structural empowerment** focuses on ensuring that appropriate processes are in place to accomplish the mission, vision, and values of the organization.
- **Exemplary professional practice** focuses on empowering nursing staff with the resources needed to provide consistent, high-quality care and demonstrate expertise in the area of nursing.
- **New knowledge, innovation and improvements** focuses on continuous learning and growth, and redesigning processes as appropriate to continuously improve patient care.
- **Empirical quality results** focuses on organizations developing systems to measure clinical outcomes related to nursing care.

Review the nursing practice for compliance prior to application, because much time and effort are involved in applying for the award. Entrance criteria include the following:

- A chief nursing officer with a Master's degree and, if the Master's is not in the field of nursing, a minimum Bachelor's degree in Nursing. The CNO must participate in the highest decision-making and strategic planning bodies.
- Nurse managers (all of whom must have a Bachelor's or Master's degree in nursing). The nurse managers are accountable for supervising all registered nurses below them.
- Nurse leaders and nurse educators all with at least a Bachelor's degree in nursing.
- The nursing administration uses ANA's standards.
- The organization has protected feedback procedures, whereby nurses can express concerns without fear of retribution.
- The organization has committed no unfair labor practices involving a nurse for 3 years prior to application.
- The organization complies with all relevant regulatory requirements.
- The organization's data collection includes nurse-sensitive indicators.

Evaluating Compliance

CPHQ Role

Documentation

The CPHQ must update documentation requirements based on changes to regulatory or accreditation standards. This means that the CPHQ must be cognizant of accreditation standards, such as those by the Joint Commission, and current regulations, such as those related to CMS or HIPAA, and monitor closely to determine if current documentation is adequate or if changes must be made. Accreditation standards require huge amounts of paperwork to demonstrate compliance, so building requirements into the system can save time when reports are due; thus, the CPHQ must consider retrieving data as well as documenting necessary information when updating. While CMS provides updates regarding most federal regulations, states may have additional requirements that must be accommodated. Changes should be made well in advance of required compliance so that staff members can become familiar with changes and problems with changes can be evaluated.

Facilitating Communication

The CPHQ's role in facilitating communication with accrediting and regulatory bodies includes:

- Understanding the preferred method of communication (electronic [email, messaging], telephone, personal contact, postal mail) and to whom or what department communication should be directed.
- Utilizing the correct format for communication.
- Keeping abreast of all changes and compliance issues that may need to be addressed.
- Maintaining open communication with administration and others who deal with compliance issues and reporting any changes or issues of concern.
- Anticipating the need for more information or clarification.
- Maintaining a timeline and monitoring activities, tracking survey and reporting dates.
- Communicating at the appropriate time.
- Consulting others about issues of concern and actively seeking input.
- Greeting and orienting surveyors to the facility and introducing them to key stakeholders.
- Preparing notes and talking points for administrators and others involved in compliance.

Survey Readiness

COORDINATING SURVEY PROCESSES

Survey processes include accreditation, licensure, and contractual requirements. The CPHQ is responsible for coordinating survey processes. The coordinator's goals are to ensure that:

- All necessary data is collected
- The proper format is used
- The most cost-efficient method is used

In some cases, electronic data sources are **incompatible**, making it impossible to transfer data, and the costs of new software can be considerable. Take a thorough inventory of all performance measures and data collected across the organization:

- Send a data inventory questionnaire to all departments, requesting information about their types of data and reasons for its collection.
- Organize the inventory results according to:
    - Core measures
    - Outcomes
    - Processes
- List definitions of the data types, storage methods, job titles of persons responsible for data collection, and legal uses of the data.
- Match a complete list of all required measures against the inventory to verify compliance. It is at this point that duplications or deficiencies should become evident.

MAINTAINING CONTINUOUS READINESS

Continuous readiness means that an organization meets or exceeds the minimum accreditation and regulatory standards at all times. The survey processes coordinator must ensure the organization is in a constant state of survey readiness through the following:

- **Identification of leadership**: Ask the governing board to identify an administrative team and clinical leaders who will assume the responsibility for and commit to continuous readiness. Identify senior leaders in each survey area, who ensure compliance. Assemble teams for quality activities to review standards and compliance.
- **Monitoring**: When the board assigns appropriate interdisciplinary teams to monitor readiness, ensure those responsible meet four times yearly to review the organization's compliance with standards. Walkabouts and self-assessments should be conducted regularly and interviews or focus groups can be used to gather information. Corrective action plans should be put into place following assessments if deficiencies are found.
- **Structure and activities**: Document the type of administrative and team structure used for survey readiness, including team activities and responsibilities.
- **Tracer methodology and performance measures**: Conduct some form of mock survey or self-assessment regularly.
- **Information and communication**: Distribute standards and guidelines to leaders for reference. Flag changes in standards. Review the surveyors' reports for the last two full surveys to determine if previous recommendations have been instituted. Communicate compliance standards to staff via corporate intranet, newsletters, and in-service training sessions.

- **Evaluation**: Assess all monitoring activities with software appropriate for finding patterns, trends, causes, and opportunities for improvement. Track specific performance measures and review them regularly.
- **Intervention**: Evaluate data to drive interventions. Schedule pre-surveys as early as possible in order to implement changes.

MAINTAINING KNOWLEDGE READINESS FOR ACCREDITATION

Knowledge readiness refers to maintaining the staff's knowledge of the most up-to-date practices, protocols and procedures of the facility that meet the accreditor's standards and core measures. Knowledge readiness can be maintained through the following:

- **Inform**: Distribute standards, explanatory material, and updates to team leaders, area leaders, and individuals involved in the accreditation or regulatory processes. Identify and apprise staff of annual changes in standards or survey processes.
- **Review**: Review previous surveys. List previous recommendations that require action. Make action plans. Review all focused survey reports and progress reports. Review previous and current performance improvement evaluation reports to ensure recommendations are implemented.
- **Identify**: Spotlight new compliance issues, such as annual National Patient Safety Goals and National Performance Goals.
- **Evaluate**: Determine the current status of all performance improvement activities and outcomes. Scrutinize supporting data to ensure it is adequate.
- **Determine**: Ascertain compliance with ethics and anti-fraud policies. Scrutinize patient safety issues and the need for changes in the patient safety program.
- **Revise**: Review and revise policies and procedures as needed, to ensure consistent standards apply organization-wide.

PRE-SURVEY PREPARATION

Pre-survey preparation involves periodic self-assessment in order to evaluate compliance with standards and to prepare for on-site surveys:

- Organize walkabouts in all departments and areas, and focus on selected standards.
- Assemble focus teams to monitor selected standards.
- List standards on a grid, with the appropriate documentation format to show compliance
- Develop a complete electronic record or binder to outline each function or standard, with necessary references.
- Delegate tasks related to recommendations.
- Document all process improvement activities with one type of form.
- Educate those involved in process improvement.
- Inform staff of compliance issues and ensure all are familiar with the survey process and their roles.
- Review personnel records for proper credentialing, records of orientation, and completeness.
- Network with other CPHQs about surveys.

USING TRACER METHODOLOGY FOR ACCREDITATION

Tracer methodology looks at the continuum of care a patient receives from admission to post-discharge.

There are three types of tracers:

- **Individual tracers** follow the patient encounter from admission to discharge, identifying potential opportunities for improvement regarding care, treatment, and services.
- **System tracers** evaluate a particular process within an organization following the results from individual tracers. Review includes identifying breakdowns in coordination or communication within a process. System tracers typically include the areas of data management, infection control, and medication management.
- **Focused tracers** identify risk or safety concerns related to care, treatment, or service and review program-specific requirements to ensure compliance.

Accreditation surveyors utilize tracer methodology when completing their assessment of an organization, so the CPHQ can test an organization's readiness by emulating the surveyors. Select a patient to trace, using his medical record as a guide. Use the experiences of this patient, as told in documents and interviews, to evaluate the processes in place at the organization. For example, the patient selected received physiotherapy, so as a mock surveyor, begin by scrutinizing:

- **Physiotherapist**: How did the PT receive the doctor's order and arrange for patient transport? How was physiotherapy administered? How was progress noted?
- **Porter**: How did the porter receive the transport request? How long did the transfer take? What route was used? What method was used to transport this patient? How was transport equipment cleaned afterwards? What do porters do if an emergency arises during transport?
- **Nurse**: How did the nurse notify the PT of the doctor's order? How did the nurse prepare the patient? How did the nurse know the therapy schedule? How did the nurse coordinate the patient's physiotherapy with other treatments? How did the nurse learn about the patient's progress?

CPHQ Practice Test #1

Want to take this practice test in an online interactive format? Check out the online resources page, which includes interactive practice questions and much more: **mometrix.com/resources719/cphq-27315**

1. Which of the following maps the expected course of interdisciplinary care for those with the same diagnosis over a specific timeframe?
   a. Algorithm
   b. Protocol
   c. Guideline
   d. Clinical pathway

2. Principles of high-reliability organizations include:
   a. Staff loyalty to the organization
   b. Constant concern with cost-effectiveness
   c. Constant concern regarding failure
   d. Routine recognition and rewards for quality service

3. Philip Crosby's (1961) quality improvement process introduced the idea of:
   a. Quality control
   b. Zero defects
   c. Quality planning
   d. Healthcare deliverables

4. A position has recently opened for a department head in human resources (HR). It is your job to select the best internal candidate to interview for the position. Which of the following candidates possesses the strongest leadership potential?
   a. An HR employee who has been with the organization for 10 years
   b. An accounting supervisor who has a perfect quality record
   c. An HR employee who mentors new hires and frequently attends voluntary training
   d. A supervisor in the maintenance department who wants to try something new

5. If conducting clinical research and selecting a probability sample of adults that includes 20 of ages 18-39, 20 of ages 40-59, and 20 of ages 60 and older, the type of sampling utilized is:
   a. Cluster sampling
   b. Systematic sampling
   c. Stratified random sampling
   d. Simple random sampling

6. If one of the hospital's strategic goals is to enhance the organization's clinical capabilities, which of the following improvement projects would have priority?
   a. Expanding the emergency department to become a trauma center
   b. Investing in updated technology, including digital tools for patients
   c. Providing educational programs for community members
   d. Entering partnerships with health systems and provider organizations

7. Team members begin to reach consensus on the rules for operation during the stage known as:
   a. Storming
   b. Forming
   c. Norming
   d. Recognition

8. A healthcare quality professional has been tasked with developing a plan to address lengths of stay at an inpatient facility. Data have shown that particular groups of patients tend to stay in the hospital longer than others due to a lack of transportation. What is the most impactful action for the healthcare quality professional to take when developing this plan?
   a. Establish partnerships with local organizations and/or develop healthcare plans to provide resources.
   b. Collaborate with clinical staff to ensure that patients are only discharged when their transportation home is confirmed.
   c. Inform patients of their expected discharge date in advance.
   d. Allow patients to determine their discharge date so that transportation accommodations can be made.

9. If the data set includes 68, 82, 86, 89, 90, 90, 91, 91, 92, 92 and 94, the median value is:
   a. 89
   b. 89.5
   c. 90
   d. 90.5

10. With primary triage, which is part of emergency preparedness, patients who are able to wait 45 to 60 minutes for care are color-coded:
    a. Red
    b. Black
    c. Green
    d. Yellow

11. Which of the following does NOT contribute to evidence-based practice in healthcare?
    a. Clinical expertise
    b. Evidence collected by expert panels
    c. Tradition
    d. Patient preferences

12. It is confirmed that a patient who sat for 30 minutes in the waiting room of your clinic was diagnosed with measles. What necessary infection-control step should be taken?
    a. Educate the patient on possible effects of the measles.
    b. Document the case in your annual clinic statistics.
    c. Train front-desk employees to recognize signs of measles.
    d. Contact all patients who may have been in the waiting room that day.

13. Medical orders for behavioral restraints for those ages 9 through 17 are time-limited to:
    a. 8 hours
    b. 6 hours
    c. 4 hours
    d. 2 hours

14. If 50 cardiac care beds generated over 100,000 cardiac alarms in a 60-day period (an average of about 33 per bed per day) resulting in excess noise and stress for patients and staff, the first step in reducing the number of alarms is to:
    a. Survey staff members for suggestions.
    b. Change the parameters for alarms.
    c. Assess the number of alarms that were critical and non-critical.
    d. Have alarms sound only at the nurse station and not at bedside.

15. Whenever possible, medication orders should be by:
    a. Weight
    b. Volume
    c. Dose
    d. Strength

16. One goal in the implementation of Lean Six Sigma practices in a hospital will be:
    a. Reduction in inventory
    b. The creation of systems for verifying orders
    c. Reduction in staff
    d. Reduction in manufacturing costs

17. As an administrator, you are planning to implement a process change that will improve patient safety throughout your organization. Who will likely play the biggest role in getting employees motivated to change?
    a. Champions
    b. Administrators
    c. New hires
    d. Team facilitators

18. A patient care team is in disagreement over new admissions procedures. What decision-making model should management use?
    a. Decision criteria
    b. Consensus
    c. Invocation
    d. Tenure influence

19. Which of the following is an example of qualitative data collection?
    a. Reviewing post-surgical infection statistics
    b. Surveying patients for satisfaction levels
    c. Analyzing employee attendance rates
    d. Collecting emergency room wait-time data

20. The main difference between a dashboard and a scorecard is that:
    a. A dashboard is only to be viewed by senior administrators.
    b. A scorecard includes performance measures from multiple departments.
    c. A dashboard only includes one measure of performance.
    d. A scorecard describes past performance, while a dashboard depicts performance in real time.

21. If a mental health patient has eloped from a locked unit when the exit was inadvertently left ajar, the initial response should be to:
    a. Contact the patient's family.
    b. Notify security and search the facility.
    c. Notify the police.
    d. Broadcast description on public intercom.

22. Which of the following are goals of the Electronic Health Record (EHR)?
    I. Guiding clinical practice
    II. Assisting with patient identification
    III. Personalizing care
    IV. Improving population health
    a. I and II
    b. I, II, IV
    c. I, II, III, IV
    d. I, III, IV

23. In a successful lean healthcare facility, the largest costs related to quality will be incurred by:
    a. Preventive efforts
    b. Internal failures
    c. Assessment programs
    d. External failures

24. When preparing data for display, which of the following may be distracting to the viewer?
    a. Font size 14 is used for text and size 16 for headings.
    b. Text is against a bright yellow background.
    c. The Verdana font is used for text.
    d. Highlighted text is underlined.

25. Physician privileges are granted by:
    a. Peers
    b. The governing board
    c. The medical board
    d. Executive leadership

26. According to the Pyramid of Evidence (Haynes), AKA the 5 S's (Studies, Syntheses, Synopses, Summaries, and Systems), which of the following would be categorized under Syntheses?
   a. Detailed description of research project
   b. Meta-analyses
   c. Case studies
   d. Concept analysis

27. Which of the following correctly describes the distinction between quality improvement and quality assurance?
   a. Quality assurance focuses on problems; quality improvement focuses on systems and processes.
   b. Quality assurance is a prospective approach; quality improvement is a retrospective approach.
   c. Quality assurance is monitored through continuous review; quality improvement is monitored through periodic audit.
   d. Quality assurance relies on the involvement of interdisciplinary teams; quality improvement relies on compliance with established standards.

28. Which of the following performance improvement models would be the best recommendation for a clinic that wants to discover the source of problems in patient care, eliminate these problems, and achieve consistently high-quality results in patient care?
   a. FOCUS
   b. Six Sigma
   c. PDCA
   d. LEAN

29. Which of the following immunizations does the CDC currently recommend for all healthcare workers who cannot demonstrate immunity?
   a. Hepatitis B
   b. Pneumococcal
   c. Herpes zoster (shingles)
   d. Meningococcal

30. As department manager, it is your job to conduct an annual performance appraisal for each employee in your department. One of your employees is exhibiting significant issues in response times for patient requests. How can you best incorporate performance improvement into the employee's performance appraisal?
   a. Incorporate punitive measures into the evaluation.
   b. Use encouraging words to help the employee improve.
   c. Set specific performance goals and a re-appraisal date.
   d. Performance improvement is not part of performance appraisal.

31. In order to allow for comparison among similar patients, mortality data is:
   a. Patient refined
   b. Risk-adjusted
   c. Excluded
   d. Aggregated

32. When carrying out failure mode and effects analysis (FMEA) to identify and correct process failure before utilization, what type of chart/diagram is used to identify each step in the process?
   a. Pareto chart
   b. Flow chart
   c. Pie chart
   d. Ishikawa (fishbone) diagram

33. The main difference between the Taguchi model of service provision and the traditional model is that:
   a. The Taguchi model identifies waste any time a process varies from its target.
   b. The traditional model is less forgiving of error.
   c. The Taguchi model is only applicable to manufacturing processes.
   d. The traditional model requires an organization with at least fifty employees.

34. The Centers for Medicare and Medicaid Services (CMS) 3-day rule requires:
   a. That beneficiaries wait up to 72 hours prior to their benefits becoming active
   b. A 3-consecutive-day inpatient hospitalization prior to admission to a skilled nursing facility
   c. A 3-day waiting period after receipt of a denial prior to appealing
   d. 72 hours spent in observation status prior to the inpatient admission being fully covered

35. A disagreement has arisen between the hospital administration and the members of one of its departments. The disagreement is in connection with the authority of the different parties involved and whether or not the administration can require the department to perform a certain task. What is the healthcare quality management professional's role in this?
   a. Review the rules establishing authority and inform the parties about how these rules apply to the department and the administration.
   b. Advise the department to respect the authority of the hospital administration and to follow its expectations for department performance.
   c. Consider the statements from both sides and participate in finding a solution that meets the expectations of both parties.
   d. Create a review board to act as a mediator between the hospital administration and the department to find an agreeable solution.

36. A health care facility has eleven wheelchairs. The likelihood that a wheelchair will be available when needed can be calculated with a(n):
   a. Binomial distribution
   b. Multinomial distribution
   c. Factorial
   d. Effects analysis

37. When facilitating quality improvement, the biggest barrier to implementation of changes is usually:
   a. Administration
   b. Staff resistance
   c. Cost constraints
   d. Time constraints

38. All of the following are roles of the healthcare quality management professional in terms of performance improvement teams EXCEPT:
    a. Directing the activities of performance improvement teams
    b. Guiding the expectations of performance improvement teams
    c. Removing members from performance improvement teams
    d. Taking part as a member of performance improvement teams

39. When making a process map as part of needs assessment, the CPHQ must map the process as:
    a. It actually takes place
    b. It should take place
    c. It will take place
    d. People report it takes place

40. During a surgical procedure, a small medical instrument was left inside a patient. The follow-up surgery to remove the instrument is an example of:
    a. Quality improvement
    b. Quality control
    c. Quality assurance
    d. Total quality

41. Which of the following reportable diseases requires a mandatory written report?
    a. Varicella (chicken pox)
    b. Influenza
    c. Pertussis
    d. Gonorrhea

42. How does the World Health Organization Surgical Safety Checklist lead to tight coupling in the operating room?
    a. It establishes universality for patients.
    b. It compartmentalizes the procedures.
    c. It establishes a clear operating room hierarchy.
    d. It closely aligns the various individuals involved in the process.

43. What is the primary role of the healthcare quality management professional regarding the integration of quality concepts within an organization?
    a. Creating training programs that inform staff members about the organization's quality concepts and the expectations for them
    b. Reviewing benchmarking data from other facilities to ensure that all standards are being met within the organization
    c. Defining the quality concepts for the organization and developing ways to incorporate these concepts into day-to-day activities
    d. Incorporating quality concepts into the employee appraisal system to reward employees who effectively apply the concepts

44. A patient had a 7-day hospitalization to treat a myocardial infarction that led to coronary artery bypass graft surgery. The patient's insurance predetermined the reimbursement available for the hospitalization and surgery after identifying the circumstances. This reimbursement method is known as:
   a. A prior authorization
   b. An episode of care
   c. The case rate
   d. Managed care

45. For a control chart monitoring the output of a process, which of the following findings indicates a need to review the process for special cause variation?
   I. 9 consecutive data points below the center line
   II. 6 consecutive increasing data points
   III. 3 non-consecutive data points that are in the outer 1/3 of the upper control limit
   IV. 1 data point that lies directly on the lower control limit
   a. I and II
   b. I and III
   c. I, II, and III
   d. I, II, III, and IV

46. If data about patients' genders are collected, these data are categorized as:
   a. Ordinal
   b. Discrete
   c. Continuous
   d. Nominal

47. If utilizing the Lean-Six Sigma approach to performance improvement, the primary focus should be on:
   a. Execution of project by project
   b. Strategic goals
   c. Cost-effectiveness
   d. Identification of errors

48. A large clinic is looking to introduce some costly changes into the facility. These changes will require careful budgeting. The healthcare quality management professional is likely to assist the facility in all of the following EXCEPT:
   a. Reviewing staff salaries to cut unnecessary expenses on benefits programs
   b. Supporting the facility in setting up a budget for effecting the changes
   c. Providing a cost analysis of the changes to ensure a satisfactory cost-return ratio
   d. Researching potentially unexpected costs to avoid going over-budget

49. Before facilitating change in a healthcare organization, it's especially important to have an understanding of the organizational:
   a. Service population
   b. Financial status
   c. Structure
   d. Culture

50. When dealing with conflict in a team, which of the following would be classified as an unconscious reactive response?
   a. Showing respect
   b. Accepting accountability
   c. Expressing feelings
   d. Blaming others

51. The type of database that is generally utilized to track such things as inventory and purchases is a(n):
   a. Relational database
   b. Operational database
   c. Hierarchical database
   d. Real-time database

52. Under tort law, a nurse who tells an uncooperative patient that he is being ridiculous and threatens to carry out a treatment on the patient against the patient's will may be charged with:
   a. Battery
   b. Assault
   c. False imprisonment
   d. Defamation of character

53. Which of the following best expresses the way a healthcare quality management professional can utilize technology for a healthcare facility's patient safety program?
   a. Research available software and assist in selecting the best software option for the facility.
   b. Work with the IT department to ensure that patient safety goals are met throughout the facility.
   c. Send out email reminders about patient safety to each department within the facility.
   d. Provide patient safety information on the facility's website for the public to review.

54. All of the following are areas of competency for Focused Professional Practice Evaluation EXCEPT:
   a. Interpersonal and communication skills
   b. Patient care
   c. Medical or clinical knowledge
   d. Documentation

55. Which of the following is the best definition of "vision" in regards to creating an organizational vision statement?
   a. The ability to see the future
   b. An ideal future state
   c. A realistic action plan for future performance
   d. An outline of future organizational purpose

56. Within the last four days, three post-surgical patients have died of pneumonia complications at a large hospital. None of the patients presented as symptomatic for pneumonia at the time of surgery. What evaluation tool should be used to help identify and resolve this issue?
   a. Epidemiological theory
   b. Performance management measures
   c. Statistical analysis
   d. Improvement measures

57. A healthcare quality management professional's responsibility toward improving patient safety includes all of the following EXCEPT:
   a. Assisting in the development of a patient safety culture throughout the organization
   b. Researching technology options for improving the current patient safety program
   c. Incorporating patient safety goals into the governance documents of the organization
   d. Informing patients at the organization about the facility's patient safety goals

58. If a review of IV medication errors finds that most errors are related to incorrectly programmed infusion pumps, the best solution is to:
   a. Provide increased training.
   b. Switch to "smart" pumps.
   c. Allow only advanced practice nurses to program pumps.
   d. Take punitive action for errors.

59. You are deeply involved in preparing an award application, and you need to survey internal subject matter experts to answer the questions needed for the application. What question would be appropriate for any survey, regardless of the department or subject?
   a. Describe your departmental approach to patient care.
   b. Describe your departmental approach to customer service.
   c. Describe your departmental approach to financial management.
   d. All of the above.

60. Considering measures of distribution, what percentage of values should be expected to fall outside of 3 deviations from the mean?
   a. 10%
   b. 5%
   c. 2%
   d. <1%

61. The shift from the triple aim to the quadruple aim includes the addition of:
   a. Provider experience
   b. Cost containment
   c. Reduction in readmissions
   d. Patient experience

62. If a reimbursement method is going to change, and a date (6 months in the future) and a grace period (an additional 3 months) have been set for implementation, the best time to begin to implement the change is:
    a. Immediately
    b. In 4 months (before implementation)
    c. In 6 months (at implementation)
    d. Before end of the grace period

63. All of the following are important elements of organizational transparency for a healthcare facility EXCEPT:
    a. Annual reports about facility costs and activities
    b. A public statement about facility values
    c. A public explanation of all activities within facility
    d. Clear information about facility partnerships

64. According to Hospital Compare, the most common overall rating for hospitals is:
    a. 1 star
    b. 2 stars
    c. 3 stars
    d. 4 stars

65. Which of the following is NOT one of the types of quality problems identified by the Institute of Medicine's National Roundtable on Health Care Quality?
    a. Misuse
    b. Abuse
    c. Overuse
    d. Underuse

66. A small city has two hospitals. The Hospital Consumer Assessment of Healthcare Providers and Systems (HCAHPS) reports show Hospital A is performing far below Hospital B in customer service. The administrators at Hospital A decide to set an organizational goal of ranking higher than Hospital B in customer service in one year. What is the most logical first step in the goal-setting process?
    a. Develop an overall goal with a breakdown of the partial goals needed to achieve the overall goal.
    b. Identify a specific and singular goal to be initially pursued.
    c. Require immediate training for all members of each department.
    d. Bring in customer service experts to evaluate and improve processes.

67. One way to create useful alignment in an organization is to:
    a. Base the assessment of each department on the same set of performance dimensions.
    b. Have each employee report to a single manager.
    c. Eliminate adverse drug events.
    d. Organize interdepartmental meetings.

68. In a large hospital setting, which of the following represents an internal customer?
   a. An admitted patient
   b. A physical therapy department assistant
   c. A medical equipment supplier
   d. A patient's family

69. If a measure appears reasonably valid to those utilizing the measure, the measure has:
   a. Construct validity
   b. Content validity
   c. Face validity
   d. Discriminant validity

70. Which one of the following serves as the best resource to extract data to drive population health improvement efforts?
   a. Patient experience surveys
   b. Electronic health record (EHR) data
   c. Value-based care performance reports
   d. United States Census Bureau

71. Following an audit by a regulatory body, what is the healthcare quality management professional's role in assisting a healthcare facility?
   a. Present the healthcare facility with the list of recommendations from the regulatory body.
   b. Review the audits from the regulatory body and research improvements to be made.
   c. Determine the source of the problems to ensure future compliance with regulations.
   d. Integrate the recommendations of the regulatory body into the facility's goals and activities.

72. The most common source of the goal statement for a tree diagram is:
   a. An affinity diagram
   b. The root cause identified by an interrelationship digraph
   c. An assignment
   d. A histogram

73. According to the Diffusion of Innovations theory (Rogers), the first stage in the spread of innovations is:
   a. Knowledge
   b. Persuasion
   c. Decision
   d. Implementation

74. Hospital X was recently ranked last in the region in the area of efficiency in transferring patients to inpatient beds. When working on process improvements, what type of data is likely to prove most helpful?
   a. Internal data
   b. Historical data
   c. Quality control data
   d. Comparative data

75. Which of the following types of charts is best for determining whether or not a process is stable?
   a. Control chart
   b. Density plot
   c. Venn chart
   d. Spline chart

76. The four basic elements of malpractice include (1) duty to use due care, (2) breach of duty, (3) damages, and (4):
   a. Causation
   b. Intent
   c. Liability
   d. Conspiracy

77. The type of power that a staff nurse obtains by closely affiliating with the unit supervisor is:
   a. Connective
   b. Coercive
   c. Legitimate
   d. Referent

78. In terms of performance measurements, which of the following is derived from a national performance system developed by Joint Commission?
   a. Consensus standards
   b. Accountability measures
   c. Continuous quality improvement
   d. Core measures

79. The CPHQ is investigating the cause(s) of a sentinel event in which a relatively stable patient with a hemorrhagic stroke was inappropriately diagnosed with an ischemic stroke after the physician failed to read the CT results correctly. The patient was admitted over night when the radiology department was short-staffed and unavailable to confirm the CT scan's result. Resulting from the misdiagnosis, the nurse administered tPA per the physician's order. The effect of tPA drastically worsened the hemorrhage, leading to the patient's death. In this case, what party may be considered liable?
   a. The physician who misdiagnosed the patient and ordered tPA
   b. The nurse who administered the tPA that ultimately lead to the patients expedited death
   c. The hospital, for not having the staff available to support this patient
   d. Nobody would be considered liable, as the patient's condition was severe and likely to result in death

80. The process of determining risk in order to proactively identify needs, outcomes, and costs is based on:
   a. Documentation and coding review
   b. Time series analysis
   c. Claims review
   d. Predictive modeling

81. A patient was discharged from the hospital following a stroke and was then readmitted several days later for a broken wrist. This is an example of a(n):
   a. All-cause readmission
   b. Risk-adjusted readmission
   c. Stratified readmission
   d. Planned readmission

82. Before construction begins on a renovation project, what assessment(s) should be completed?
   a. Risk management
   b. Quality measures
   c. Life safety and infection control
   d. Medical equipment and materials

83. The healthcare quality management professional typically participates in all of the following processes EXCEPT:
   a. Medical record review
   b. Peer review
   c. Governance review
   d. Service specific review

84. In a control chart, the central line represents the:
   a. The average of data points
   b. The time period
   c. The count/rate
   d. The lower limit of data

85. A hospital uses the same labels for all of its prescriptions, but these labels do not fit on the smallest container, so employees must cut and paste the labels in a special way in order to fill the prescription. This is an example of:
   a. Overproduction
   b. Queuing
   c. Work-in-progress
   d. Extra processing

86. Which of the following methods of statistical analysis is appropriate to determine if there is a statistically significant difference between the means of two groups?
   a. Chi-squared
   b. T-test
   c. Regression analysis
   d. Range

87. The primary component of a life safety management program is:
   a. Fire prevention plan
   b. Information backup plan
   c. Utilities management
   d. Staffing protocols

88. **The Baldrige Performance Excellence Program Health Care Criteria remark on the importance of measurement and analysis of data. What can be the downside of a heavy performance data focus?**
   a. Managers can get tunnel vision and overlook non-measured errors and issues.
   b. Data far above the national standard can result in inflated self-opinion.
   c. Data far below the national standard can result in depression and despondency.
   d. Hospitals with high data scores are held to impossibly high standards.

89. **What is the primary role of the healthcare quality management professional in terms of consultant activity within a healthcare facility?**
   a. Monitoring all consultant activity to ensure that it meets the standards for quality and patient safety
   b. Researching the history of consultant activity by contacting other facilities and requesting information
   c. Communicating to the consultant all information about facility expectations for patient treatment
   d. Assembling a review team to ensure that the consultant follows facility procedures and policies

90. **On review of emergency department records to evaluate patient safety issues, which of the following suggests medical overuse?**
   a. RICE therapy routinely prescribed for muscle strains
   b. CT ordered for head trauma in 40% of cases
   c. Opioid prescriptions limited to 7-day supply
   d. Antibiotics prescribed for cough in 85% of cases

91. **What four types of quality measures are pay-for-performance programs usually based on?**
   a. Costs, outcomes, timeliness, and best practices
   b. Performance, costs, outcomes, and patient experience
   c. Performance, outcomes, patient experience, and structure/technology
   d. Patient experience, outcomes, costs, and timeliness

92. **The most important characteristic of the controls in a case-control study is that they are:**
   a. Drawn from a random pool of patients
   b. Identical to the cases in every respect except for the presence of the targeted condition
   c. Available for frequent observation
   d. Literate

93. **When creating a control chart, the control limits are set at:**
   a. 1 *sigma* (standard deviation) above and 1 *sigma* below center line
   b. 2 *sigmas* above and 2 *sigmas* below center line
   c. 3 *sigmas* above and 3 *sigmas* below center line
   d. 4 *sigmas* above and 4 *sigmas* below center line

94. Regarding employee performance within a healthcare facility, the healthcare quality management professional's primary role includes all of the following EXCEPT:
   a. Assembling comparative data to measure employee performance
   b. Applying employee performance improvement to the facility's evaluation system
   c. Creating a program that recognizes employee performance improvement activities
   d. Identifying positive employee activity and indicating employees appropriate for promotion

95. The process of risk management for the healthcare quality management professional includes all of the following EXCEPT:
   a. Identification of risk
   b. Analysis of effects
   c. Reporting of incidents
   d. Prevention of risk

96. The healthcare quality management professional can expect to contribute to the development of survey processes for all of the following EXCEPT:
   a. Accreditation
   b. Safety policy
   c. Governance
   d. Licensure

97. A root cause analysis of inpatient suicides would be most likely to discover problems with:
   a. Staffing levels
   b. Staff orientation
   c. The physical environment
   d. The risk assessment of the patient

98. Which component of decision-making typically receives much less time than it deserves?
   a. Framing
   b. Gathering information
   c. Drawing conclusions
   d. Voting

99. If a hospital is part of a provider network but contracts with providers (such as anesthesiologists) who are not in the plan's network, resulting in multiple complaints of "surprise bills," the hospital should:
   a. Leave the matter to legal counsel.
   b. Notify patients in advance of estimated costs.
   c. Utilize only in-network providers.
   d. Ignore complaints as part of doing business.

100. If the process improvement team leader assigns a team facilitator, that individual's role is to:
   a. Schedule meetings.
   b. Manage conflicts and group dynamics.
   c. Record information.
   d. Coordinate data collection.

101. The goal of population health aligns most closely with:
   a. Health equity
   b. Quality improvement
   c. Risk prevention
   d. Patient compliance

102. A healthcare facility has been very pleased with the results of the performance improvement teams that the healthcare quality management professional facilitated. Additionally, the facility has noticed that employee productivity has improved, and the facility would like to quantify this improvement. How might the healthcare quality management professional assist in this process?
   a. Develop a plan for adding the performance improvement findings and activities to employee evaluations.
   b. Create a rewards hierarchy for each employee who participated in a performance improvement team.
   c. Generate an annual bonus plan that provides an incentive to employees who participated on a performance improvement team.
   d. Assist the facility in sending personalized messages to all employees who were part of a performance improvement team.

103. A hospital-wide set of professional standards is important because it:
   a. Reduces the waste of time and resources
   b. Eliminates bottlenecks
   c. Encourages duplication
   d. Minimizes the need for communication

104. Which of the following is most likely to be identified as a process champion?
   a. An individual with a particular interest in performance improvement
   b. A team leader who is involved in supervising a team
   c. The chairman of the board of directors
   d. The supervisor of a clinical unit

105. Before instituting organization-wide utilization of SBAR for hand-offs and transitions of care, the CPHQ should initially:
   a. Survey the staff.
   b. Provide guidelines and training.
   c. Mandate a date for implementation.
   d. Advise staff to research SBAR.

106. Juran's "quality trilogy" comprises quality planning, quality improvement, and quality:
   a. Evaluation
   b. Product
   c. Outcomes
   d. Control

107. Most quality problems in healthcare are the result of:
    a. Lack of compassion
    b. Lack of resources
    c. Disorganization
    d. Ignorance

108. All of the following represent federally-mandated patient rights in the United States EXCEPT:
    a. Right to informed consent for medical treatment
    b. Right to maintain the privacy of medical records
    c. Rights to obtain a copy of medical records
    d. Right to receive healthcare services

109. If an outbreak of *Clostridioides difficile* has occurred resulting in multiple cases of severe diarrhea in hospitalized patients and staff members on one unit, the initial infection control efforts should be aimed at:
    a. Isolating patients with the infection
    b. Closing the unit for disinfection
    c. Penalizing staff members
    d. Hand washing procedures

110. One disadvantage of using separate scorecards for financial and customer satisfaction data is that:
    a. Administrators are likely to overvalue the financial information.
    b. Employees will become confused.
    c. There is likely to be more resource waste.
    d. It requires special training.

111. In terms of performance measurements, which of the following represents a visual summary of performance data from within an organization?
    a. Dashboard
    b. Performance productivity report
    c. Outcome data
    d. Surveyor report

112. Clinic A has just completed six months of customer satisfaction surveys. Excellence in performance has been appropriately recognized. Now complaints must be analyzed and somehow quantified. What method would be most effective in the complaint analysis process?
    a. Sort surveys into separate folders.
    b. Create a taxonomy for coding complaints.
    c. Address complaints one at a time.
    d. Match complaints with performance issues.

113. Which of the following is vastly different from the others?
    a. SIPOC
    b. DMAIC
    c. PDCA
    d. PDSA

114. In a typical hospital, approximately what percentage of errors is reported?
   a. Less than 10
   b. Between 25 and 50
   c. 75
   d. Between 80 and 90

115. Following the results from a large-scale performance improvement study that has reviewed all departments of a healthcare facility, the healthcare quality management professional's primary role is to:
   a. Review the results of the performance improvement study.
   b. Apply the results of the performance improvement study.
   c. Disseminate information about the study for employee education.
   d. Evaluate the overall effectiveness of the performance improvement study.

116. Which of the following is absolutely essential for the leader of an effective performance improvement team?
   a. "Type A" personality
   b. Charisma and persuasion
   c. Modeling target behaviors
   d. Extended tenure with the organization

117. The administration of a hospital has discovered that a lack of communication among different hospital departments has led to overspending and unnecessary errors in patient care. The administration has asked the healthcare quality management professional to assemble a team that can improve department communication and address the problems. What type of team would be most useful for this task?
   a. Cross-functional team
   b. Management team
   c. Intradisciplinary team
   d. Emergency response team

118. A healthcare quality management professional's responsibility regarding information management in a healthcare facility generally includes all of the following EXCEPT:
   a. Define data.
   b. Collect data.
   c. Summarize data.
   d. Qualify data.

119. When developing a survey, the questions should be arranged:
   a. At random
   b. According to categories
   c. From specific to general
   d. From general to specific

120. Which of the following poses a potential risk of infant/child abduction?
   a. Fire alarms disengage door locks.
   b. Mothers and infants have identical ID bands.
   c. Employees wear ID badges with color photos.
   d. There is one public entry to the nursery area.

121. To ensure that food service areas of the hospital are in compliance with safety regulations, records of cleaning should be documented every:
   a. 8 hours
   b. 24 hours
   c. Week
   d. Month

122. If a patient satisfaction survey covers topics clearly related to issues of patient satisfaction, the type of validity the survey has is:
   a. Criterion validity
   b. Discriminant validity
   c. Content validity
   d. Convergent validity

123. All of the following are aspects of the Voice of the Customer (VOC) tool EXCEPT:
   a. Hierarchical structure
   b. Perception of performance
   c. Priorities
   d. Cost

124. Which of the following is the primary role of the healthcare quality management professional in terms of committee meetings?
   a. Lead the committee meeting as an objective participant.
   b. Review the topics to be discussed in the committee meeting.
   c. Organize and maintain the information from the committee meeting.
   d. Disseminate information from the committee meeting to different departments.

125. A healthcare facility has asked the healthcare quality management professional to assist in the performance improvement process for the facility. All of the following are steps the healthcare quality management professional can take to get started on this process EXCEPT:
   a. Establishing strategic goals for the performance improvement teams
   b. Developing performance improvement activities for the facility to utilize
   c. Reviewing the performance improvement results for future application
   d. Creating projects for the performance improvement teams to complete

126. Which one of the following options is NOT an effective strategy for healthcare organizations to use to address health disparities?
   a. Providing cultural competency training to all providers
   b. Hiring providers from the medical school within the community
   c. Partnering with organizations in the local community
   d. Opening locations in underserved communities

127. Under tort law, if a patient states his intention of signing himself out of the hospital against medical advice and a nurse prevents the patient, who is of sound mind and poses no risk to self or others, from leaving, the nurse may be charged with:
   a. Assault
   b. False imprisonment
   c. Battery
   d. Kidnapping

128. A complete history and physical examination should be completed on an inpatient with no recent history of care within:
   a. 6 hours
   b. 12 hours
   c. 18 hours
   d. 24 hours

129. A department within a healthcare facility has consistently been going over-budget. The department claims that its budget is not sufficient for its required activities, while the facility claims that the department is spending excessively and needs to reduce costs. What is the role of the healthcare quality management professional in this situation?
   a. Assist the department in setting up a manageable budget and working within it.
   b. Communicate between the department and the facility to ensure a satisfactory agreement.
   c. Establish for the department a clear budget that reflects the facility's expectations.
   d. Review the activities of the department to see whether there is anywhere to cut costs.

130. When conducting a serious adverse/sentinel event investigation, which type of analysis may be used proactively to identify potential problems that may occur in order to determine which part of a process most requires change?
   a. Root cause analysis (RCA)
   b. Strength, Weakness, Opportunity, Threats (SWOT) analysis
   c. Gap analysis
   d. Failure Mode Effect Analysis (FMEA)

131. When creating a flow chart, the geometric figure (decision icon) used to represent areas in a process where an evaluation or decision must be made is the:
   a. Square
   b. Rectangle
   c. Diamond shape
   d. Oval

132. Which of the following professional liability sources does not require establishing a standard, as the act of negligence is clear?
   a. Vicarious liability
   b. Ostensible agency
   c. *Res ipsa loquitur*
   d. Corporate liability

133. The protocol for ordering a medication should be:
   a. The same every time
   b. Customizable
   c. Adaptable to verbal or written situations
   d. Dependent on inventory

134. The pathology department of Hospital A is up for a service-specific review. What documents should be considered as part of this review?
   a. General policies and procedures for the hospital
   b. Employee work history and performance statistics
   c. Specific policies and procedures for pathology
   d. All of the above

135. Material safety data sheets (MDSSs) must be available:
   a. On file in Administration
   b. In each department
   c. Upon request
   d. At locations of hazardous materials

136. If the organization's overall staff turnover rate exceeds the benchmark (<6%) set by the organization, the next step should be to:
   a. Analyze the rate by job class.
   b. Survey all staff regarding job satisfaction.
   c. Develop a strategy for retention.
   d. Carry out a salary comparison study.

137. The first stage of strategic planning involves:
   a. External and internal environment assessment
   b. Review of mission, goals, and objectives
   c. Identifying a list of possible strategies
   d. Conducting a cost-effectiveness analysis

138. If a power outage delayed surgeries when the backup power system failed, this would be classified as a:
   a. Common cause variation
   b. Special cause variation
   c. Random variation
   d. Direct variation

139. Which of the following is a method used to measure instrument reliability?
   a. Internal consistency measures
   b. Scale reliability coefficient
   c. Instrumental calculation
   d. Test-retest reliability coefficient

140. Which of the following groups is least likely to report errors?
   a. Primary care physicians
   b. Support staff
   c. Independent contractors
   d. Nurses

Answer Key and Explanations for Test #1

1. D. A clinical pathway maps the expected course of interdisciplinary care for those with the same diagnosis over a specific timeframe, such as the number of days of anticipated hospitalization for a patient. The pathway indicates the expected nursing outcomes for each day and the interventions needed. The clinical pathway is based on average lengths of stay. Deviations from the pathway should be immediately addressed through team meetings and changes made to improve outcomes.

2. C: Principles of high-reliability organizations include:

- Constant concern regarding failure, constantly on alert.
- Focus on promoting organizational resilience, responding quickly to problems and errors.
- Attention to operations and allowing some autonomy to solve problems.
- Adequate communication with documentation standards adhered to.
- Promotion of culture or safety with reporting of problems rewarded.

3. B: Philip Crosby's (1961) quality improvement process introduced the idea of zero defects. Crosby's quality process is based on:

- Conformance to requirements/standards.
- Prevention efforts rather than appraisal.
- Zero defects as the performance standard.
- Measurement is the price of nonconformance.

Crosby believed that 3 things were essential in promoting quality: determination, education, and implementation.

4. C: An employee with experience in the field who has emotional intelligence (demonstrated by mentoring new hires) and a quest for new knowledge shows excellent leadership potential. Years of experience and perfect quality records do not necessarily translate into strong leadership; therefore, individuals who have already displayed leadership qualities regardless of title should be given priority.

5. C: If conducting clinical research and selecting a probability sample of adults that includes 20 of ages 18-39, 20 of ages 40-59, and 20 of ages 60 and older, the type of sampling utilized is stratified random sampling (a form of probability sampling). This type of sampling is indicated when one or more variables in the sampling frame are essential. Variables utilized for sampling may include age, gender, diagnosis, healthcare provider, type of organization/institution, type of procedure, and geographical location.

6. A: If one of the hospitals strategic goals is to enhance the organization's clinical capabilities, then the improvement project that would have priority is expanding the emergency department to become a trauma center. Trauma centers include specialized staff, including surgeons and other physicians, who are trained to deal with severe injuries, such as gunshot wounds and traumatic brain injuries. Trauma centers are often part of the emergency department and allow trauma patients to be treated rather than stabilized and transferred.

7. C: Team members begin to reach consensus on the rules for operation during the stage known as norming. That is, they begin to establish group norms. The four general stages of group behavior are forming (when the group first comes together), storming (when differences are aired and arguments occur), norming, and performing (when the group accomplishes its tasks). Some sociologists include a final recognition stage, in which group members acknowledge the steps that have been taken and resolve to modify their group behavior in the future.

8. A: In this situation, it is evident that social determinants of health are playing a role in preventing patients from timely discharge. With this in mind, the healthcare quality professional's best next step is to establish partnerships or nurture existing partnerships with organizations and develop healthcare plans that provide resources, such as transportation, to patients. Although informing patients of their expected discharge date in advance is also a good strategy, it does not address the root cause of the problem.

9. C: It the data set includes 68, 82, 86, 89, 90, 90, 91, 91, 92, 92 and 94, the median value is 90. When the data are placed in ascending order, the date point in the middle is the median. Median may be more accurate than mean because of outliers. For example, the mean of the 11 numbers above is 965/11 = 87.7. However, only 3 number fall below that average while 8 numbers fall above. The outlier of 68 gives an inaccurate picture of the data while the median (90) is a more accurate reflection.

10. D: Yellow. Primary triage:

- P1—Red: Immediate care needed for urgent systemic life-threatening conditions, such as airway/breathing problems, severe bleeding, severe burns (especially with breathing problems), decreased mental status, shock, and severe medical problems, Glasgow Coma Score ≤13.
- P2—Yellow: Delayed care and able to wait 45-60 minutes for treatment for burns (without breathing problems), multiple bone/joint injuries, back and/or spinal cord injuries (unless in respiratory distress).
- P3—Green: Hold, able to wait hours for treatment of minor injuries, "walking injured."
- P4—Black: Deceased.

11. C: Tradition does not contribute to evidence-based practice in healthcare. The evidence-based practice movement consists of a renewed emphasis on scientific rigor and empirical data. The preferences of patients are considered, but the primary determinant of intervention and therapy is the evidence from research studies and the experience of practitioners. Traditional methods of therapy may be investigated to determine their efficacy, but they are not used for sentimental or cultural reasons. In addition to clinical expertise, evidence, and patient preferences, evidence-based practice devises therapies based on patient history and the availability of resources.

12. D: The most important infection-control step in this situation, after reporting the confirmation to the local health jurisdiction immediately, would be to contact all patients who may have been in the waiting room that day. The measles are a highly communicable and dangerous disease; therefore every patient that was exposed to the carrier must be assessed and informed of possible consequences of this exposure.

13. D: Medical orders for behavioral restraints for individuals ages 9 through 17 are time-limited to two hours, while for those under 9 are limited to one hour, and for those 18 and over, to four hours. Behavioral restraints should be avoided if at all possible and removed as soon as the patient reaches criteria for discontinuation. Patients younger than 17 must be reassessed for continued need for restraints at least every 4 hours, and those 18 and over, every 8 hours.

14. C. If 50 cardiac care beds generated over 100,000 cardiac alarms in a 60-day period (an average of about 33 per bed per day) resulting in excess noise and stress for patients and staff, the first step in reducing the number of alarms is to assess the number of alarms that were critical and non-critical. The results should be evaluated and a determination made regarding which non-critical alarms can be eliminated. Single-use sensors (such as for ECG) should be changed on a routine basis to prevent alarms when they disengage.

15. C: Whenever possible, medication orders should be by dose. This is the most important variable related to medication, and the one which has the most relevance to the products actually used by the patient. Medication orders that are classified by weight, volume, or strength are often confusing to pharmacists. Moreover, several different unit systems (e.g., metric or SI) may be used, so there is a greater risk of error. To reduce the possibility of mistakes, healthcare facilities should standardize the protocol for medication orders.

16. A: One goal in the implementation of Lean Six Sigma practices in a hospital will be a reduction in inventory. The developers of this organizational philosophy assert that there are numerous costs associated with maintaining a large inventory. Essentially, they believe that it is impossible to operate at peak efficiency while maintaining a large store of products and resources. Although many people believe that the implementation of Lean Six Sigma practices will lead to reductions in staff and manufacturing costs, this is not necessarily the case.

17. A: Champions are respected "key players" in the organization and will therefore be most likely to play a big role in getting employees motivated to change. Their respect within the organization will make their opinion and input heard. While administrators have formal power through their title, that is not necessarily a motivational tool. Team facilitators are focused more on process facilitation than motivation.

18. A: Decision criteria is a decision-making model that explores all options equally and gives unorthodox or unpopular options a fair chance, even when they are under dispute. Consensus is not the best choice because this approach often reduces decisions to options that everyone likes and discounts the unorthodox or unpopular options that could be appropriate and viable.

19. B: Surveying patients regarding satisfaction results in qualitative feedback because the answers are more subjective and perspective-dependent than quantitative data. The other options are incorrect because they produce quantitative data that is objective and not qualitative in nature.

20. D: The main difference between a dashboard and a scorecard is that a scorecard describes past performance, while a dashboard depicts performance in real time. Indeed, a dashboard is so-called because it is analogous to the dashboard of a car, which delivers current metrics. Dashboards are better for making quick adjustments, whereas scorecards are better at providing a comprehensive, clear-eyed view of performance over the recent past.

21. B. If a mental health patient has eloped from a locked unit when the exit was inadvertently left open, the initial response should be to notify security and search the facility. Security should monitor exits and review video footage if available. If the patient is not located, then the patient's home should be called as that is typically a patient's destination. Whether or not to call the police depends on the patient's decision-making capacity and risk to self or others.

22. D: The Electronic Health Record (EHR) has four main goals, to guide clinical practice, interconnect clinicians, personalize care and improve population health. The EHR was not established with the goal of assisting with patient identification. This is more appropriately addressed with the implementation of barcode scanning.

23. A: In a successful lean healthcare facility, the largest costs related to quality will be incurred by preventive efforts. Indeed, a lean facility is likely to spend much more than another facility on prevention. A lean facility saves money by reducing errors and eliminating waste. Moreover, prevention programs in a lean facility tend to be more efficient and targeted. Over time, a lean healthcare facility may be able to phase out certain elements of prevention.

24. B: When preparing data for display, text against a bright color (such as yellow) may be distracting to the viewer. It is harder for the eyes to process text from an illuminated screen than from paper, and this can result in blurring if the font is too small (less than 12) or if print fonts (such as Times New Roman) are utilized instead of digital fonts designed for the web, such as Verdana and Lucida Sans/Grande. Text should be broken up into small paragraphs and underlining used to highlight text rather than bolding or italics.

25. B: Physician privileges are granted by the governing board. The governing board may include executive leadership, such as a CFO, but typically includes additional representatives such as physicians. Peers often evaluate physicians during peer review but do not have input during privileging. Medical boards license and discipline physicians, but do not have authority to grant privileges within an organization.

26. B: According to the Pyramid of Evidence (Haynes), AKA the 5 S's, a meta-analysis is categorized under syntheses. Pyramid:

- Studies (base): Qualitative studies, quantitative studies, case studies, and concept analyses.
- Syntheses: Systematic reviews, meta-analyses, literature reviews, integrative reviews.
- Synopses: Brief descriptions of research projects and studies.
- Summaries: More detailed descriptions of research projects and studies.
- Systems (point): EHRs integrated with practice guidelines.

Studies and syntheses carry the most weight when developing evidence-based guidelines and pathways.

27. A: Quality assurance is a component of quality improvement and is a process that focuses on monitoring problem areas or individuals against established policies and procedures for compliance. Quality improvement is both a prospective and retrospective process that focuses on systems and the processes involved that need to be addressed for positive change. With quality improvement, there is a need for continuous review, while quality assurance relies on periodic inspections.

28. B: Six Sigma is recommended as a performance improvement model that enables an organization to reduce problems and, more importantly, achieve consistency in results. The other performance improvement models, FOCUS, PDCA, and LEAN, offer variations of problem identification and reduction, but only Six Sigma specifically focuses on generating consistently good results.

29. A: Immunizations that the CDC currently recommends for all healthcare workers includes hepatitis B and influenza (annually). Other recommended immunizations include:

- MMR (measles, mumps, rubella): Two-dose series with the second immunization at least 28 days after the first for those born after 1957 and those born before 1957 without proof of immunity.
- Varicella (chicken pox): Two doses, four weeks apart.

- Tdap (tetanus, diphtheria, and pertussis): One time with tetanus (TD) booster every 10 years.
- Meningococcal: One dose.

30. C: The best way to incorporate performance improvement concepts into an employee appraisal is through specific performance goals and a set re-appraisal date. A and B are incorrect because they are not concrete performance improvement techniques. Performance improvement is an integral part of a performance appraisal; therefore, it is appropriate to address this issue through the proposed performance improvement goals.

31. B: Mortality data should be risk-adjusted to allow for appropriate comparison among groups of patients. Risk adjustment is a statistical process that takes into consideration additional factors that may contribute to patient outcomes. For example, an elderly patient with several chronic conditions and a history of cancer likely has a higher expected mortality when experiencing a stroke than a teenager experiencing a stroke with no risk factors or morbidities. In order to compare the two outcomes equitably, risk adjustment is required.

32. B: When carrying out failure mode and effects analysis (FMEA) to identify and correct process failure before utilization, the type of chart that is used to identify each step in the process is a flow chart. In the flow chart, each step in the process is numbered consecutively and each sub-step lettered consecutively. This chart then is used when brainstorming each step and sub-step to determine if they have the potential for failure.

33. A: The main difference between the Taguchi model of service provision and the traditional model is that the Taguchi model identifies waste any time a process deviates from its target. In the traditional model, on the other hand, a process is considered optimal so long as it falls within a broad set of specifications. The Taguchi model brings a sense of perfectionism to service provision. It establishes ideal conditions, and then notes any areas in which the operation falls short. For this reason, it is better at informing quality improvement efforts.

34. B: The CMS 3-day rule requires beneficiaries to spend 3 consecutive days in inpatient care prior to qualifying for coverage for admission to a skilled nursing facility. The day of discharge is not counted in this calculation, nor is any time prior to actually being admitted, such as time spent in the emergency department or in observation status. Beneficiaries may receive a waiver that removes the inpatient stay requirement prior to qualifying for skilled nursing facility coverage, but the beneficiary must still meet the level of care.

35. A: In terms of a dispute, the healthcare quality management professional's role is only to understand how the lines of authority are drawn and to present this information to the parties involved. She should not take sides in any way, making answer choice B incorrect. Additionally, she is not responsible for mediating or even finding a solution (unless asked specifically to do so). The role in this case is largely one of providing the information and allowing the parties to consider it.

36. A: The likelihood that a wheelchair will be available when needed can be calculated with a binomial distribution. A binomial distribution is appropriate for illustrating probabilities when there are two possible events. In this case, the two possible events are that a wheelchair will either be available or not. A healthcare facility could use binomial distributions to determine the likelihood of a wheelchair being available for any given number of wheelchairs. This would be a way to determine the optimal number of wheelchairs for the facility to keep on hand.

37. B: When facilitating quality improvement, the biggest barrier to implementation of changes is usually staff resistance to change. People develop a sense of security with familiarity, and new approaches, even though they may be demonstrably better, can result in anxiety and insecurity. Some people may feel that the changes suggests that they were less than competent before, and others may resent the time and effort needed to learn new skills or ways of doing things.

38. C: The healthcare quality management professional is not necessarily responsible for removing members from the performance improvement teams. He might recommend removal, but the decision is likely to come from a higher source. The healthcare quality management professional is, however, expected to direct the activities, guide the expectations, and take part as a member of performance improvement teams.

39. A: When making a process map as part of needs assessment, the CPHQ must map the process as it actually takes place, not as it should or will with changes. This means, that the process should be mapped during direct observations and surveys, taking note of any work-arounds or shortcuts that are utilized. People often inaccurately report steps in a process. The process map should include times, such as the time needed to obtain supplies, and the complete cycle time from beginning to end.

40. C: Quality assurance is a focus on outputs or quality after the point of production, including any corrective actions necessary to optimize post-production quality, as in the surgery performed to remove the instrument left in the patient. A, B, and D are incorrect because they refer to quality processes that take place on different levels and are not corrective in the way that quality assurance is.

41. D: Gonorrhea, along with many other diseases such as syphilis, TB, and malaria, are reportable diseases that require a written report. State laws may vary slightly in reporting requirements, which are based on CDC guidelines. Different types of reporting are required, depending on the disease. Some, including rubeola and pertussis, must be reported by telephone. Only totals rather than individual cases must be reported for some diseases, such as varicella, mumps, and influenza.

42. D: The World Health Organization Surgical Safety Checklist leads to tight coupling in the operating room by closely aligning the various individuals involved in the surgical process. This checklist has three parts: sign in, time out, and sign out. Each part includes a checklist that must be read out loud to the surgical team to ensure that all important elements of the surgical procedure have been reviewed and agreed upon by the entire team, from patient allergies, to surgical site confirmation, anesthesia preparation, and patient risks.

43. C: The primary role of the healthcare quality management professional for the integration of quality concepts is in defining the quality concepts for the organization and developing ways to incorporate these concepts into day-to-day activities. The creation of training programs, the review of benchmarking data, and the incorporation of quality concepts into the employee appraisal system all fall under this larger category, but all are too specific to encompass the full role.

44. B: An episode of care involves a series of services provided to a patient for a specified period of time, including the assessment, treatment, and ongoing management of the condition at hand. It involves an all-inclusive payment model in which reimbursement is calculated to include all services received by the patient. This type of payment model ensures alignment by encouraging providers to focus on achieving positive outcomes for patients rather than identifying ways to increase revenue through higher volume.

45. A: I and II. A review for special cause variation can be indicated by any of several triggers. NAHQ recognizes five:

- Any data point that falls outside of the 3σ control limits (a data point on the control limit does not qualify)
- 2 out of 3 consecutive data points that fall outside the 2σ line (in the outer third of the control limit)
- 8 consecutive points on one side of the center line
- 6 or more consecutive increasing or decreasing data points
- 15 or more consecutive data points within 1σ of the center line (should be reviewed due to the likelihood that the control limits are not well calibrated)

46. D: If data about patients' genders are collected these data are categorized as nominal data. Nominal data are based on the lowest level of measurement because they basically just separate data into categories—in this case male, female, or other (gender non-specific, transgender). Other nominal data may include ethnicity, job title, and blood type. Nominal data cannot be treated mathematically. For example, it's impossible to calculate the average gender, only the average number of people in one gender.

47. B: If utilizing the Lean-Six Sigma approach (which combines Six Sigma with "lean" thinking) to performance improvement, the primary focus should be on strategic goals. The program aims to provide continuous learning and rapid change to reduce error and waste. Characteristics include:

- Long term goals and strategies for 1- to 3-year periods.
- Performance improvement as the underlying belief system.
- Cost reduction through quality increase.
- Incorporation of improvement methodology, such as DMAIC, PDCA, or other methods.

48. A: It is not necessarily the responsibility of the healthcare quality management professional to make cuts in staff salaries. What is more, it is unlikely that a healthcare facility would dip into staff salaries to find money for a program. The healthcare quality management professional is, however, responsible for supporting the facility in setting up a budget, providing a cost analysis to ensure a good cost-return ratio, and researching potentially unexpected costs.

49. D: Before facilitating change in a healthcare organization, it's especially important to have an understanding of the organizational culture, which comprises attitudes, beliefs, behaviors, and shared assumptions. Different basic types of organizational cultures include:

- Stable learning cultures where people exercise skills and advance over time.
- Independent cultures in which people have valued skills that are easily transferable to other organizations.
- Group cultures in which there is strong identification and emphasis on seniority.
- Insecure cultures with frequent staff layoffs and reorganization.

50. D: An unconscious reactive response, such as blaming others, is based on feelings rather than rational thought or recognition of those feelings. Other unconscious reactive responses include making unreasonable demands on others, usually in response to anxiety or distress, or passing unfair judgments on others. With conscious reactive responses, the person recognizes and acknowledges personal feelings and thoughts, accepts accountability, and shows respect and compassion for others.

51. B: An operational database is generally utilized to track such things as inventory, purchases, patient information, and all financial transactions. Hierarchical databases are organized in a tree or parent-child formation with one piece of information connected to many (one-to-many), but in descending order only (not many-to-one). Relational databases are built on a multiple table structure with each individual item on a table having a unique identifier. Relational databases allow both one-to-many and many-to-one relationships. Real-time databases are used for rapidly changing data, such as stock market reports.

52. B: Under tort law, a nurse who tells an uncooperative patient that he is being ridiculous and threatens to carry out a treatment on the patient against the patient's will may be charged with assault. Any threat to touch or harm a patient in some way without the patient's permission may be considered assault. Battery, on the other hand, is actually carrying out the act, such as (in this case) carrying out the treatment.

53. A: Utilizing technology for a patient safety program typically involves researching available software and assisting in selecting the best software option for the facility. Working with the IT department might be part of this process, but it is only one part and too narrow to describe the full responsibility of the healthcare quality management professional in the situation. Sending out email reminders and providing patient safety information on the facility's website, again, might be part of the process, but both fail to embrace the full scope of applying technology for a patient safety program.

54. D: The Focused Professional Practice Evaluation (FPPE) has six areas of competency: patient care, medical or clinical knowledge, practice-based learning and improvement, interpersonal and communication skills, professionalism, and systems-based practice. While documentation is an important part of provider practice, it is not a stand-alone area of competency tested for FPPE.

55. B: In the creation of an organizational vision statement, vision is a description—realistic or not—of an ideal future state. This description of an ideal future state gives shape to the goals of an organization. A vision statement does not involve detailed descriptions about the specific actions necessary for bringing the vision to fruition.

56. A: Epidemiological theory is used to identify the source and cause of an issue or anomaly, which is perfect for the surgical complications represented in this question. The other tools are used to quantify data points of a health care organization or to examine processes that can contribute to improvement. Prior to establishing improvement measures for this particular instance, the epidemiological theory will help identify the source of the issue around which improvement measures can focus.

57. D: Again, there is not necessarily a need to inform patients directly about the specific patient safety goals of the organization. The fact that the organization is committed to patient safety should be information enough. The healthcare quality management professional does have the responsibility to assist in the development of a patient safety culture within the organization, research technology options for improving the patient safety program, and incorporate patient safety goals within governance documents of the organization.

58. B: If a review of medication errors finds that most errors are related to incorrectly programmed infusion pumps, the best solution is to switch to "smart" pumps. Standard infusion pumps deliver whatever is programmed while smart pumps have access to drug libraries appropriate for different units and preset drug parameters that limit the ability of the programmer to make errors because alerts occur if the drug is outside of these parameters (dosage too high or too low, infusion too fast).

59. B: Every department can and should answer survey questions describing their approach to customer service. Departmental approaches to patient care and financial management may also be relevant but are dependent on the department and/or subject, therefore are not the appropriate answer.

60. D: Almost all values fall within 3 deviations of the mean. Less than 1% should fall beyond that. Standard deviation (square root of the variance) shows how data is distributed above and below the mean in equally measured distances. Usually about 68% of the data points fall within the first standard deviation, 95% within the first two deviations, and 99.7% within the first three deviations. If the data points are spread out over a large range, then the standard deviation is higher than if the data points are closer to the mean.

61. A: As the healthcare industry has evolved, the triple aim has transitioned into the quadruple aim. The triple aim focuses on improving the health of populations, reducing per capita cost, and improving the experience of care. The quadruple aim adds a fourth factor for consideration, which involves improving the work-life experience for providers.

62. A: If a reimbursement method is going to change and a date (6 months in the future) and a grace period (an additional 3 months) have been set for implementation, the best time to begin to implement the change is immediately. Implementation may require programming, staff training, data collection, and other activities, so preparation should begin when notice is received so that the organization is ready at the time of implementation.

63. C: Organizational transparency does not necessarily include a public explanation of all activities within the facility. That could rapidly prove to be a logistical—as well as a public relations—nightmare. Organizational transparency tends to be more standard: an annual report about facility costs and activities, a public statement about facility values, and clear information about facility partnerships (i.e., who has a stake in activities, and who does not; whether there is any potential for a conflict of interests).

64. C: According to Hospital Compare, the most common overall rating for hospitals is 3 stars (32% of hospitals that provide enough data to be rated). 14% percent of hospitals receive the highest 5-star rating, and only 6% received the lowest 1-star rating. The ratings are based on scores for five different types of measures: mortality, safety of care, readmission, patient experience, and timely and effective care. The hospital scores are compared with national averages and information on the site indicates if the hospital is above, at, or below national averages.

65. B: Abuse is not one of the types of quality problems identified by the Institute of Medicine's National Roundtable on Health Care Quality. Misuse, overuse, and underuse are the three most common problems; they also represent three sources of waste in health care. The National Roundtable on Health Care Quality was significant because it asserted that the provision of health care services can be assessed with scientific precision. This was a major step towards incorporating business and manufacturing productivity systems in health care.

66. A: When undertaking a goal-setting process, the best first step is to develop an overall goal that is broken down into smaller partial goals that must be met in order to achieve the overall goal. B is wrong because it doesn't account for how the overall goal will be obtained. C and D are incorrect because they are reactive steps, not proactive steps.

67. A: One way to create useful alignment in an organization is to base the assessment of each department on the same set of performance dimensions. In lean organizations, alignment is valued because it brings clarity. When all of the departments in an organization are evaluated according to the same dimensions of performance, each employee will be able to assess his or her own department as well as the other departments. Also, it will be easy for administrators to compare the performances of all the departments.

68. B: A physical therapy department assistant is an internal customer because he or she works within the organizational structure. Inpatients, medical equipment suppliers and patient family members all represent external customers whom rely on and/or utilize the health care organization and product.

69. C: Face validity: The measure appears reasonably valid to those utilizing the measure. Construct validity: The scale measures that which it is intended to measure. Content validity: The scale measures the range of meanings/items that make up the concept. Discriminant validity: Degree of difference that occurs in the results if the measure is utilized in different settings.

70. B: The electronic health record (EHR) is a great resource to use for identifying data to drive population health improvement efforts. Although the data can sometimes be unstructured and siloed, the healthcare quality professional can use analytics to identify areas of opportunity within this information. EHR data contain information regarding patient history (medical and social) and demographics, claims, encounters, and medications, among many other facts—all of which help provide a well-rounded picture of the patient experience. Patient experience surveys and reports from value-based care contracts may also reflect information-gathering opportunities, but their scope is limited and may not be reflective of the entire patient population.

71. D: Following an audit, the healthcare quality management professional should take steps to integrate the results of the audit into the facility's goals and activities. Answer choices A, B, and C reflect individual steps in this larger goal, but each is too narrow to be the best option.

72. B: The most common source of the goal statement for a tree diagram is the root cause identified by an interrelationship digraph. Interrelationship digraphs outline all of the factors that influence an issue, and then isolate the one factor that has the most influence. This factor is known as the root cause. On a tree diagram, the root cause will be entered first as the goal statement. Then, the diagram will depict the operations that must be performed to achieve the goal statement.

73. A: According to the Diffusion of Innovations theory (Rogers), the first stage in the spread of innovation is knowledge. Stages:

- Knowledge: Becoming aware of an innovation and its purpose and function. May be obtained through various methods, such as literature research, conference attendance, educational classes.
- Persuasion: Developing positive or negative attitudes.
- Decision: Making a commitment, which may result in adoption or not and continuing the innovation or not.
- Implementation: Putting the innovation into action.
- Confirmation: Evaluating.

74. D: Comparative data would prove most helpful in improving the processes at Hospital X. By comparing their data and processes with those of higher-ranked medical facilities, process improvement solutions could be derived. A and B are incorrect because internal data, whether historical or contemporary, will not help identify the reasons for the last place ranking and will not help improve processes. C is wrong because quality control data is another internal measure that will only compare the existing processes with established internal standards.

75. A: A control chart is most useful for seeing the changes in a process, and thus for determining whether or not a process is stable. It uses an x- and y-axis and a horizontal line that represents an average around which points of progress are charted to determine the processes' stability (closeness to the average) or instability. A density plot has the same focus as a histogram (examining the distribution of data over a period of time), using smoothed and rounded lines rather than bars. A Venn chart is used to visually represent commonalities and differences between various items. A spline chart is similar to a line graph, but the line used to connect the points plotted is curved as a representation of how data changes over the course of time. While stability may be inferred from a spline chart, it is not its primary focus.

76. A: The four basic elements of malpractice include:

- Duty to use due care: Failure to meet standards set by law, contract, or standard practice.
- Breach of duty: An act of omission or commission.
- Damages: Harm that results, may be physical, emotional, or financial.
- Causation: Evidence that the breach of duty resulted in the damages.

In order to receive judgment for a plaintiff (the complainant), all four of these elements of malpractice must be proven.

77. D: The type of power that a staff nurse obtains by closely affiliating with the unit supervisor is referent power. That is, others may feel that the personal or professional connection that exists might allow the person to influence supervisorial decisions. The degree of referent power that the nurse has is a direct reflection of the degree of respect (or fear) that the staff members hold for the supervisor. Referent power may be respected or resented.

78. D: The term "core measures" is derived from a national performance system developed by Joint Commission. These measures are the foundation upon which the Joint Commission standardizes their performance evaluation of healthcare facilities for the sake of accreditation. The Joint Commission also established accountability measures, but these are considered quality measures that fall within the Joint Commission's performance measures (there are also non-accountability measures). Consensus standards are part of the National Quality Forum's performance measures. Continuous quality improvement (CQI) is a method and philosophy of quality control and quality assurance used across the healthcare industry and other organizations.

79. A: In this scenario, the physician may be considered liable for the patient's expedited death as a result of their misdiagnosis, due to the fact that any reasonable physician working in the emergency department would be expected to appropriately differentiate between an ischemic stroke and hemorrhagic stroke on a CT scan, and choose treatment appropriately. While it is possible for a nurse to have noticed the misdiagnosis and the dangerous treatment selection, it is not within the nurse's scope to interpret imaging results, and therefore they were staying within their scope by appropriately executing the doctor's orders. While the hospital being short staffed, particularly at night, is a concern that the CPHQ should address through process improvement measures, the hospital would not be considered liable in this situation because doctors are expected to be able to interpret radiology reports. The patient was stable on admission; therefore, the severity of their condition did not necessarily presume an end result of death.

80. D: The process of determining risk to proactively identify needs, outcomes, and costs is based on the process of predictive modeling. Predictive modeling analyzes data from disparate sources, reviewing trends and patterns that may indicate potential future events. Data that are typically reviewed to establish a predictive model include, but are not limited to, claims data, pharmacy data,

EHR data, lab test results, and imaging results. The purpose of this review is to determine potential risks and provide an opportunity to proactively intervene to avoid poor outcomes. A review of claims, documentation, and coding data would be considered in this circumstance, but this information would be used to target the predictive modeling process.

81. A: All-cause readmissions occur when a patient has an unplanned acute readmission for any cause within 30 days. Although some readmissions are unavoidable, data suggest that some readmissions are due to poor discharge planning and/or care coordination after discharge. Healthcare quality professionals should support interdisciplinary teams to ensure that transitions of care are monitored appropriately and an effective, ongoing care plan is established to reduce the risk of readmission.

82. C: Before construction begins on a renovation project, life safety and infection control assessments should be completed to evaluate the risk. The construction may negatively impact life safety codes if, for example, it increases the risk that a fire may occur. Additionally, if the construction generates dust, this can pose a considerable risk of infection to vulnerable patients. Also, if there is water damage, spores may be released, so the flow of air between the construction site and the rest of the facility must be carefully assessed.

83. C: The healthcare quality management professional's job entails participation in a medical record review, peer review, and service specific review. It does not typically involve participation in a review of the facility's governance, which is determined by a higher authority.

84. A: In a control chart, the central line represents the average of the data points. The x-axis represents the time period used (days, months, years, decades) while the y-axis represents the rate or count and the data points represent the actual values. Additionally, there is an upper control limit, a line representing +3 standard deviations from the mean and a lower control limit, a line representing -3 standard deviations from the mean.

85. D: This scenario is an example of extra processing. Extra processing is anathema to the philosophy of lean. Whenever a lean manager spots a situation like the one in this example, he will immediately work to resolve it. In this case, the hospital would be wise to adopt a labeling system that is appropriate for all of its containers. In addition to the obvious creation of more work, the extra processing described here may encourage medication errors.

86. B: The T-test is the method of statistical analysis appropriate to determine if there is a statistically significant difference between the means of two groups. The chi-square test is a means of establishing if a variance in categorical data (as opposed to numerical data) is of statistical significance. Regression analysis is used to evaluate the type of data sets found in a scattergram, so it compares the relationship between two variables to determine if the relationship correlates. Range is the distance from the highest to the lowest number.

87. A: The primary component of a life safety management program is a fire prevention plan. Fire prevention should be addressed during initial construction and outfitting of all facilities as well as during ongoing operations. Standards for fire prevention efforts are set by the National Fire Protection Association. All fire detection and fire-fighting equipment must be inspected and tested in accordance with the Life Safety Code. The plan must include a fire response plan and outline training and fire drills.

88. A: The downside of a heavy data focus can be tunnel vision by managers, which can lead to oversight of non-measured errors. While data is a good starting point for measuring performance and quality improvement efforts, it is not the only indicator of success or failure. In combination with data should be comparative efforts to external benchmarks, climate surveys and contextual support.

89. A: In this situation, the healthcare quality management professional is responsible for monitoring all consultant activity to ensure that it meets standards for quality and patient safety. Answer choices B, C, and D reflect potential elements of this responsibility (researching the history of consultant activity, communicating expectations to consultants, and assembling a review team to ensure consultants fulfill expectations), but none of these options encompass the role in full.

90. D: Because most coughs result from a viral infection for which antibiotics have no use, prescribing antibiotics for 85% of cases of cough is an indication of medical overuse that could lead to complications, such as *Clostridioides difficile* infection. Medical overuse, including ordering of multiple unnecessary tests (often done as a defensive measure out of fear of malpractice suits), increases the cost of care and often has little benefit for the patient.

91. C: Pay-for-performance programs are usually based on four types of quality measures:

- Performance: Based on carrying out practices demonstrated to improve health outcomes.
- Outcomes: Based on achieving positive outcomes (but does not always consider social or other variables that the healthcare provider cannot control).
- Patient experience (satisfaction): Based on patient's perceptions of care received and their satisfaction.
- Structures/Technology: Based on facilities and equipment used for care, and may reward some types of upgrades, such as an upgrade to an electronic health record.

92. B: The most important characteristic of the controls in a case-control study is that they are identical to the cases in every respect except for the presence of the targeted condition. Otherwise, there are too many variables that could skew the results of the study. It is not necessary for the controls to be drawn from a random pool of patients. On the contrary, researchers will frequently need to exercise extreme care in the selection of controls. Many studies do not require frequent observation, and very few require the controls to be literate.

93. C: When creating a control chart, the control limits are set 3 *sigmas* (standard deviations) above and 3 *sigmas* below the center line. Each *sigma* away from the centerline is one zone (zones A, B, and C above and below). The center line represents the mean value of the historical data. Most plotted data should fall between the control limits. As data are entered, data points that fall outside of the control limits or data points that do not show normal variation (bell curve) are considered out-of-control.

94. D: The healthcare quality management professional is not responsible for recommending specific employees for promotion. (In some cases, this might be appropriate, but it is not necessarily part of her expectations.) The healthcare quality management professional, however, is responsible for assembling comparative data to measure employee performance, applying employee performance improvement to the facility evaluation system, and creating a program that recognizes employee performance improvement activities.

95. C: The healthcare quality management professional is responsible for the following, in terms of risk management: identifying the risk, analyzing the effects of the risk, and preventing the risk. These responsibilities do not necessarily include the responsibility of reporting an incident of risk; that may or may not apply, depending on the source of the risk. (It should be noted, however, that the healthcare quality management professional is responsible for reviewing the incident report about the risk; of course, this is not the same as actually reporting an incident of risk.)

96. C: The healthcare quality management professional contributes to the development of survey processes for accreditation, safety policy, and licensure. He does not necessarily get involved with survey processes for governance, unless specifically required to do so.

97. D: A root cause analysis of inpatient suicides would be most likely to discover problems with the risk assessment of the patient. It is critical to ensure that there is a standard risk assessment utilized by trained staff and policies in place to determine precautions necessary for patient safety. Failure to properly assess a patient leads to an increased risk for sentinel events, such as suicide. Staffing levels, staff orientation, and the physical environment may also contribute to suicide, but these components are directly linked to the outcome of timely risk assessments conducted with at risk patients.

98. A: Framing is the element of decision-making that receives much less time than it deserves. Framing is the process of organizing the question to be decided. It entails listing the possible sources of information and prioritizing the decision-making process. Research suggests that groups tend to spend about five percent of the entire decision-making process on framing when they should spend about 20 percent on it. If a decision is framed well, the subsequent parts of the decision-making process will proceed with relative ease.

99. B: Public perception of a hospital is important, and patients should not receive "surprise bills." Patients should be notified in advance when out-of-network providers are used and given estimates of cost before service is provided. Patients should also be provided information about alternatives if they are available. While state laws vary, patients may be able to file a complaint through the state's consumer protection agencies if they did not receive advance notice about out-of-network costs.

100. B: If the process improvement team leader assigns a team facilitator, that individual's role is to manage conflicts and group dynamics. The team facilitator should be very familiar with the process improvement process as well as the target process or processes for the team and should ensure that the process improvement process is carried out effectively. The facilitator may also serve in the role of coach and/or mentor for other team members and serve as a consultant or advisor.

101. A: The goal of population health is to improve health outcomes and the quality of care for groups of individuals while containing costs. This may be achieved through focused efforts on quality improvement initiatives, risk prevention, and/or ensuring patient compliance; however, health equity is the term that most closely aligns with the overarching goal of population health. Health equity is a term that is used to describe the attainment of the highest level of health for individuals, and it ensures that everyone has an equal opportunity to do so through addressing social, economic, and behavioral barriers to optimal health.

102. A: The healthcare quality management professional has the option of developing a plan for incorporating performance improvement findings into employee evaluations. She does not, however, have the authority to create a rewards hierarchy or generate an annual bonus plan for employees. Additionally, the option for sending out personalized messages to employees might be a thoughtful gesture, but it hardly meets the facility's goal of quantifying the performance improvement team results.

103. A: A hospital-wide set of professional standards is important because it reduces the waste of time and resources. As much as possible, healthcare facilities should standardize professional behavior in every department in order to eliminate confusion and reduce inefficient behavior. In some cases, the adoption of universal professional standards will reduce the need for communication, but this is not a necessary consequence. Similarly, it may be that standardization will decrease the number of bottlenecks, though again, this is not inevitable.

104. A: Regardless of the individual's position, a process champion is one who has a particular interest in performance improvement and often actively seeks ways to improve processes and may, in fact, lead a process improvement team. Process champions provide an important role in influencing others, as resistance to change is common. Identifying key process champions throughout an organization and enlisting their assistance is an important step in facilitating change.

105. B: As with any changes in procedures or policies, the staff should be provided detailed guidelines and training of each element of SBAR as well as worksheets they can use to organize information. Elements include:

- Situation: Name, age, MD, diagnosis.
- Background: Brief medical history, co-morbidities, review of lab tests, current therapy, IV's, VS, pain, special needs, educational needs, discharge plans.
- Assessment: Review of systems, lines, tubes, and drains, completed tasks, needed tasks, future procedures.
- Recommendations: Review plan of care, medications, precautions (restraints, falls), treatments, wound care.

106. D: Juran, who specialized in quality management, believed that quality was both income-oriented and cost-oriented because quality usually costs less in the long-term and enhances income. Juran's "quality trilogy" comprises:

- Quality planning: Identify customers and their needs and developing products/services to meet those needs.
- Quality improvement: Developing processes that allow optimal production of the product/service.
- Quality control: Ensure the process can produce the product/service.

107. C: Most quality problems in health care are the result of disorganization. In a way, this fact is uplifting, because it suggests that improving quality may not require hiring new employees or purchasing large amounts of new equipment. However, reorganizing processes to achieve superior quality and efficiency can take many years.

108. D: There is no federally mandated right to healthcare services for people in the United States. There are other statutes —such as the law that forbids emergency rooms from turning away people without insurance— but the federal government does not guarantee to people that they have the right to receive healthcare services. The other rights listed (right to informed consent, right to privacy, right to a copy of medical records) are all protected at the federal level.

109. A: If an outbreak *Clostridioides* difficile has occurred resulting in multiple cases of severe diarrhea in hospitalized patients and staff members on one unit, the initial infection control efforts should be aimed at isolating the individual infected to minimize exposure to staff and other patients. Next, hand washing procedures should be initiated with signs posted to indicate contact precautions. The C. diff spores are very resistant and can survive for long periods on environmental surfaces. They are most often spread from one patient to another through contaminated hands. Older patients and those on long-term antibiotics are especially at risk.

110. A: One disadvantage of using separate scorecards for financial and customer satisfaction data is that administrators are likely to overvalue the financial information. Even when customer satisfaction is the avowed top priority of an organization, financial concerns nevertheless attract disproportionate attention. For this reason, administrators are encouraged to place all of the important pieces of data on the same scorecard.

111. A: The dashboard represents a digital summary of performance data from within an organization through the use of various charts, graphs, and tables on a single screen. It provides the viewer with a snapshot of the current status of an organization and can be updated as frequently as the organization desires. Performance productivity reports are far more detailed and thorough, including all data on performance measures, and require skilled analysis in order to be understood and applied to performance improvement efforts. Outcome data is just a single type of data that is included in an organization's collection of performance data. The surveyor report results from the survey process and provides a starting point from which performance measures are assessed and modified in order to address the needs of an organization.

112. B: The most effective way to analyze large numbers of complaints is through the creation of a taxonomy for coding complaints because it helps classify and organize complaints in a logical way that lends itself well to analysis.

113. A: SIPOC (suppliers, inputs, process, outputs, customers) is different from the other three acronyms, which are sequential programs for quality improvement. SIPOC, on the other hand, is a form of diagram that enables Six Sigma practitioners to identify the important components of process improvement and determine both internal and external customer needs. DMAIC (define, measure, analyze, improve, control) is a general structure for eliminating defects. Similarly, PDCA (plan, do, check, act) and PDSA (plan, do, study, act) are structures for the improvement of processes.

114. A: In a typical hospital, less than ten percent of errors are reported. Many hospital managers are surprised by this statistic, because the number of reported errors can seem large. However, healthcare facilities often have unclear or relaxed reporting policies. Part-time employees and independent contractors are much less likely to report errors. Unfortunately, the failure to report errors has negative consequences far beyond the point at which the specific error occurs. The best healthcare facilities establish mandatory error-reporting programs with an emphasis on being nonjudgmental and accepting of inevitable human error.

115. B: Immediately following a performance improvement study, the primary role of the healthcare quality management professional is simple: begin applying the results of the study to the facility. Reviewing the results is important, but this does not necessarily create needed action. Disseminating information about the study is useful, but it depends entirely on the nature of the study and whether or not employees need to know about it directly. Evaluating the overall effectiveness of the study should be part of the follow-up task, but again the primary focus should be on applying the results.

116. C: The leader of a performance improvement team must model target behaviors above all else in order to set the example for team members. Type A personalities may lead to strong leaders, but can often cross into authoritarian leadership, which is not often appropriate. Charisma and persuasion help a leader motivate team members, but must have a proper foundation and target. Therefore, those characteristics alone do not assume effective leadership. Tenure may demonstrate seniority on a company ladder, but also does not necessarily correlate with effective leadership.

117. A: The key here is the need for a team that can find ways to improve communication among the different departments. This type of team would need to be cross-functional (also referred to as multi-disciplinary or interdisciplinary), because it would be composed of people from the different departments who would then be delegated to communicate with one another and pass on the communication to others within their respective departments. A management team, as the name implies, is led by a manager. In the case of creating a team to improve communication across departments, it would be important that the members be those of non-management positions. An intradisciplinary team consists of members from a single specialty or department, and therefore would not be appropriate to address a problem that spans across departments. Emergency response teams (also known as task force teams) are assembled to address specific emergencies. While communication is critical, it would not be considered an emergency, and therefore would not require an emergency response team to be addressed.

118. D: The word "qualify" has a variety of meanings, one of which is "modify." The healthcare quality management professional certainly does not have the authority to modify data. He does, however, have the responsibility to define, collect, and summarize data.

119. D: When developing a survey, the questions should be arranged from general to specific because general questions ("Did you use laboratory services?") are less intimidating than specific ("Did you experience excessive wait time with laboratory services?"). Therefore, if a survey begins with general statements, the customer is more likely to begin and then complete the survey. The format of questions should be consistent throughout the survey and clearly stated without ambiguities that may be misunderstood.

120. A: For safety reasons, fire alarms routinely disengage door locks, but this poses a potential risk of infant/child abduction as a kidnapper may trigger the alarm in order to gain entrance. If the fire alarm sounds, then personnel must monitor entrances and exits until the children are safely evacuated or the alarm stops and locks re-engage. Areas with infants and children should have only one public entry that is within view of the nurse station and is monitored, such as by video.

121. B: To ensure that food service areas of the hospital (such as the kitchen and food storage areas) are in compliance with safety regulations, records of cleaning should be documented every 24 hours. Documentation includes recording temperatures of food and refrigerators as well as water temperature for dishwashers. All foods received in the kitchen must be properly dated, and storage must be in rodent-proof containers to prevent any contamination. The type of disinfection used must be documented.

122. C: If a patient satisfaction survey covers topics clearly related to issues of patient satisfaction, the type of validity the survey has is content validity. Discriminant validity is the degree of difference that occurs in the results if the measure is utilized in different settings. Criterion validity is the degree to which the scale correlates with another reliable scale. Convergent validity is the degree to which the scale shows a correlation between related item, such as wait time and satisfaction with service.

123. D: The Voice of the Customer (VOC) tool is used when introducing a new process, service, or product and can help healthcare quality professionals understand customer preferences. The four aspects of the VOC tool are customer perceptions of performance, customer needs, hierarchical structure, and priorities. Cost is a factor typically considered by customers but is not included in the VOC assessment tool.

124. C: For committee meetings, the healthcare quality management professional should be involved in organizing and maintaining the information from the meetings; this information might include the minutes from the meetings or any reports presented at the meetings. The healthcare quality management professional does not need to lead the meetings or disseminate information from meetings to the departments. It should also be noted that the activity of reviewing topics from the meeting is likely to fall under the larger role of organizing and maintaining meeting information.

125. C: The performance improvement results will be available after the performance improvement process has begun. So, it makes no sense to review the results as a part of getting started on the performance improvement process: there are not yet any results to review. The healthcare quality management professional can, however, establish strategic goals, develop performance improvement activities, and create projects for the performance improvement teams.

126. B: Healthcare organizations are positioned to make a positive impact on health disparities by developing strategies that address the root cause of inequity. Some of the ways in which healthcare organizations can meaningfully address health disparities are through providing cultural competency training to providers, collaborating with local organizations to provide resources such as transportation and food, and opening locations in underserved communities to improve access. It is also important for healthcare organizations to ensure that they are hiring a diverse and representative group of providers to serve the community. Although hiring providers from the medical school within the community is a great start to ensuring that the onboarded providers are familiar with the local culture and its unique needs, limiting hiring solely to the local community misses the mark strategically. Additionally, a well-balanced staff from various backgrounds would be better suited to address widespread health disparities.

127. B: Under tort law, if a patient states his intention of signing himself out of the hospital against medical advice and a nurse prevents the patient, who is of sound mind and poses no risk to self or others, from leaving, the nurse may be charged with false imprisonment. False imprisonment occurs if the patient is physically prevented from leaving, such as with restraints or locked doors, or led to believe that he is not allowed to leave.

128. D: A complete history and physical examination should be completed on an inpatient with no recent history of care within 24 hours of admission. If the patient has had a history and physical completed in the 30 days prior to admission, only an update is required, but it should also be completed within 24 hours. The nursing assessment should be completed as well within 24 hours as it is the basis for the care plan. A functional assessment should be carried out along with the nursing assessment within the 24-hour timeframe.

129. A: The primary role of the healthcare quality management professional in this situation would be to assist the department in setting up a manageable budget and working within it. Answer choices B, C, and D indicate parts of this process (communicating between the department and the facility, establishing a clear budget for the department, and reviewing the department's activities for ways to cut costs), but none of them summarizes the full responsibility of the healthcare quality management professional.

130. D: Failure Mode and Effects Analysis (FMEA) may be used proactively to identify potential problems and failures in order to determine which part of a process most requires change.. FMEA is often used to correct problems in a process prior to utilization. Steps to FMEA include:

19. Defining: outlining the process in detail.
20. Creating a team: ad hoc team of those involved in the process or with expertise.

21. Describing: numbered flow chart describes each step and sub-step.
22. Brainstorming: analyzing each step/sub-step for potential failures.

131. C: When creating a flow chart, the geometric figure (decision icon) used to represent areas in a process where an evaluation or decision must be made is the diamond shape. Other commonly used shapes include:

- Rectangle: Represents a process.
- Circle: Connects from one area of the flowchart to another (such as at the edge of a page to another page). Usually numbered; so, for example, number 1 then connects to number 2.
- Oval: Represents the end of a process.
- Lines: Show the progression of the process.

132. C: *Res ipsa loquitur* means "the thing speaks for itself" and is a type of professional liability that indicates clear negligence. Corporate liability, vicarious liability and ostensible agency are additional professional liability sources explored when determining claims in enterprise risk management. Corporate liability acknowledges that an organization owes a duty to its patients. Vicarious liability acknowledges that there is an indirect responsibility for the acts of another person, such as an employee. Ostensible agency acknowledges that organizations are typically not held liable due to the actions of an independent contractor, however, this can change depending on the specific circumstances.

133. A: The protocol for ordering medication should be the same every time. Medication errors are among the most common and most preventable in a healthcare facility. One way to reduce these errors is to standardize the prescription process. Many healthcare facilities achieve a drastic reduction in medication errors by forbidding verbal orders. In any case, the protocol for ordering a medication should not be customizable, as this is likely to create confusion and lead to error.

134. C: A service-specific review of the pathology department would cover specific policies and procedures for pathology. General policies and procedures and employee work history and performance are not relevant in a service-specific review of the pathology department.

135. D: Material safety data sheet (MDSSs) must be available at locations of hazardous materials. The MDSS should outline safety procedures and any potential hazards. MDSS must identify the chemicals, explain their characteristics (such as boiling point), outline fire/explosion hazards and any reactivity as well as health hazards. Personal protective equipment needed for handling must be outlined and any special precaution, such as for handling, transportation, or storage.

136. A: If the organization's overall staff turnover rate exceeds the benchmark (<6%) set by the organization, the next step should be to analyze the rate by job class. If, for example, the data is 9% staff turnover in nursing and 4% to 6% in other job classes, then strategies for retention need to be focused on nursing rather than on the other job classes. At this point, surveys and interviews should be carried out to obtain more data about nursing and focus groups formed.

137. B: In HQ Solutions' seven-step model, Step 1 is to define and formulate goals (aligned with mission/vision). Steps 2–3 involve assessing the external then internal environments as outlined below:

- External: A broad analysis should include review of the political climate, economic standing, demographic factors, and technology. Additionally, the competition (such as other hospitals in the area) should be assessed and the likely impact of strategic planning initiatives on this competition.
- Internal: This analysis should cover all aspects of an organization, including resources in terms of buildings, technology, and resources (human and financial).

After these steps, strategy can be formulated.

138. B: If a power outage delayed surgeries when the backup power system failed, this would be classified as a special cause variation. Special cause variations are random and cannot be predicted and generally don't require major system modification. The cause is usually easy to identify. With common cause variations, on the other hand, the variations are inherent to the process. For example, medications scheduled for 8 AM may be administered in a 30- minute window (15 minutes before and after) because of normal variations in work load, and narrowing this window may be quite difficult.

139. D: Test-retest reliability coefficient is a method used to measure instrument reliability. If information is unlikely to change, a retest of the same material should render the same results if the test is administered to the same individuals at different times. If the results vary, then the test lacks reliability and must be reassessed. If test-retest involves memory retrievable (such as a test of learned content); however, some degradation is expected because of limitations in short-term memory.

140. C: Independent contractors are the group least likely to report errors. In part, this is because they have the least personal interest in the success of the health care facility. Also, an independent contractor is more likely to view her employment as tenuous, and is therefore more nervous about admitting mistakes. A system that explicitly avoids punishing those who report will improve the incidence of error reporting among independent contractors.

CPHQ Practice Tests #2, #3 and #4

To take these additional CPHQ practice tests, visit our online resources page:
mometrix.com/resources719/cphq-27315

How to Overcome Test Anxiety

Just the thought of taking a test is enough to make most people a little nervous. A test is an important event that can have a long-term impact on your future, so it's important to take it seriously and it's natural to feel anxious about performing well. But just because anxiety is normal, that doesn't mean that it's helpful in test taking, or that you should simply accept it as part of your life. Anxiety can have a variety of effects. These effects can be mild, like making you feel slightly nervous, or severe, like blocking your ability to focus or remember even a simple detail.

If you experience test anxiety—whether severe or mild—it's important to know how to beat it. To discover this, first you need to understand what causes test anxiety.

Causes of Test Anxiety

While we often think of anxiety as an uncontrollable emotional state, it can actually be caused by simple, practical things. One of the most common causes of test anxiety is that a person does not feel adequately prepared for their test. This feeling can be the result of many different issues such as poor study habits or lack of organization, but the most common culprit is time management. Starting to study too late, failing to organize your study time to cover all of the material, or being distracted while you study will mean that you're not well prepared for the test. This may lead to cramming the night before, which will cause you to be physically and mentally exhausted for the test. Poor time management also contributes to feelings of stress, fear, and hopelessness as you realize you are not well prepared but don't know what to do about it.

Other times, test anxiety is not related to your preparation for the test but comes from unresolved fear. This may be a past failure on a test, or poor performance on tests in general. It may come from comparing yourself to others who seem to be performing better or from the stress of living up to expectations. Anxiety may be driven by fears of the future—how failure on this test would affect your educational and career goals. These fears are often completely irrational, but they can still negatively impact your test performance.

Elements of Test Anxiety

As mentioned earlier, test anxiety is considered to be an emotional state, but it has physical and mental components as well. Sometimes you may not even realize that you are suffering from test anxiety until you notice the physical symptoms. These can include trembling hands, rapid heartbeat, sweating, nausea, and tense muscles. Extreme anxiety may lead to fainting or vomiting. Obviously, any of these symptoms can have a negative impact on testing. It is important to recognize them as soon as they begin to occur so that you can address the problem before it damages your performance.

The mental components of test anxiety include trouble focusing and inability to remember learned information. During a test, your mind is on high alert, which can help you recall information and stay focused for an extended period of time. However, anxiety interferes with your mind's natural processes, causing you to blank out, even on the questions you know well. The strain of testing during anxiety makes it difficult to stay focused, especially on a test that may take several hours. Extreme anxiety can take a huge mental toll, making it difficult not only to recall test information but even to understand the test questions or pull your thoughts together.

Effects of Test Anxiety

Test anxiety is like a disease—if left untreated, it will get progressively worse. Anxiety leads to poor performance, and this reinforces the feelings of fear and failure, which in turn lead to poor performances on subsequent tests. It can grow from a mild nervousness to a crippling condition. If allowed to progress, test anxiety can have a big impact on your schooling, and consequently on your future.

Test anxiety can spread to other parts of your life. Anxiety on tests can become anxiety in any stressful situation, and blanking on a test can turn into panicking in a job situation. But fortunately, you don't have to let anxiety rule your testing and determine your grades. There are a number of relatively simple steps you can take to move past anxiety and function normally on a test and in the rest of life.

Physical Steps for Beating Test Anxiety

While test anxiety is a serious problem, the good news is that it can be overcome. It doesn't have to control your ability to think and remember information. While it may take time, you can begin taking steps today to beat anxiety.

Just as your first hint that you may be struggling with anxiety comes from the physical symptoms, the first step to treating it is also physical. Rest is crucial for having a clear, strong mind. If you are tired, it is much easier to give in to anxiety. But if you establish good sleep habits, your body and mind will be ready to perform optimally, without the strain of exhaustion. Additionally, sleeping well helps you to retain information better, so you're more likely to recall the answers when you see the test questions.

Getting good sleep means more than going to bed on time. It's important to allow your brain time to relax. Take study breaks from time to time so it doesn't get overworked, and don't study right before bed. Take time to rest your mind before trying to rest your body, or you may find it difficult to fall asleep.

Along with sleep, other aspects of physical health are important in preparing for a test. Good nutrition is vital for good brain function. Sugary foods and drinks may give a burst of energy but this burst is followed by a crash, both physically and emotionally. Instead, fuel your body with protein and vitamin-rich foods.

Also, drink plenty of water. Dehydration can lead to headaches and exhaustion, especially if your brain is already under stress from the rigors of the test. Particularly if your test is a long one, drink water during the breaks. And if possible, take an energy-boosting snack to eat between sections.

Along with sleep and diet, a third important part of physical health is exercise. Maintaining a steady workout schedule is helpful, but even taking 5-minute study breaks to walk can help get your blood pumping faster and clear your head. Exercise also releases endorphins, which contribute to a positive feeling and can help combat test anxiety.

When you nurture your physical health, you are also contributing to your mental health. If your body is healthy, your mind is much more likely to be healthy as well. So take time to rest, nourish your body with healthy food and water, and get moving as much as possible. Taking these physical steps will make you stronger and more able to take the mental steps necessary to overcome test anxiety.

Mental Steps for Beating Test Anxiety

Working on the mental side of test anxiety can be more challenging, but as with the physical side, there are clear steps you can take to overcome it. As mentioned earlier, test anxiety often stems from lack of preparation, so the obvious solution is to prepare for the test. Effective studying may be the most important weapon you have for beating test anxiety, but you can and should employ several other mental tools to combat fear.

First, boost your confidence by reminding yourself of past success—tests or projects that you aced. If you're putting as much effort into preparing for this test as you did for those, there's no reason you should expect to fail here. Work hard to prepare; then trust your preparation.

Second, surround yourself with encouraging people. It can be helpful to find a study group, but be sure that the people you're around will encourage a positive attitude. If you spend time with others who are anxious or cynical, this will only contribute to your own anxiety. Look for others who are motivated to study hard from a desire to succeed, not from a fear of failure.

Third, reward yourself. A test is physically and mentally tiring, even without anxiety, and it can be helpful to have something to look forward to. Plan an activity following the test, regardless of the outcome, such as going to a movie or getting ice cream.

When you are taking the test, if you find yourself beginning to feel anxious, remind yourself that you know the material. Visualize successfully completing the test. Then take a few deep, relaxing breaths and return to it. Work through the questions carefully but with confidence, knowing that you are capable of succeeding.

Developing a healthy mental approach to test taking will also aid in other areas of life. Test anxiety affects more than just the actual test—it can be damaging to your mental health and even contribute to depression. It's important to beat test anxiety before it becomes a problem for more than testing.

Study Strategy

Being prepared for the test is necessary to combat anxiety, but what does being prepared look like? You may study for hours on end and still not feel prepared. What you need is a strategy for test prep. The next few pages outline our recommended steps to help you plan out and conquer the challenge of preparation.

STEP 1: SCOPE OUT THE TEST

Learn everything you can about the format (multiple choice, essay, etc.) and what will be on the test. Gather any study materials, course outlines, or sample exams that may be available. Not only will this help you to prepare, but knowing what to expect can help to alleviate test anxiety.

STEP 2: MAP OUT THE MATERIAL

Look through the textbook or study guide and make note of how many chapters or sections it has. Then divide these over the time you have. For example, if a book has 15 chapters and you have five days to study, you need to cover three chapters each day. Even better, if you have the time, leave an extra day at the end for overall review after you have gone through the material in depth.

If time is limited, you may need to prioritize the material. Look through it and make note of which sections you think you already have a good grasp on, and which need review. While you are studying, skim quickly through the familiar sections and take more time on the challenging parts.

Write out your plan so you don't get lost as you go. Having a written plan also helps you feel more in control of the study, so anxiety is less likely to arise from feeling overwhelmed at the amount to cover.

STEP 3: GATHER YOUR TOOLS

Decide what study method works best for you. Do you prefer to highlight in the book as you study and then go back over the highlighted portions? Or do you type out notes of the important information? Or is it helpful to make flashcards that you can carry with you? Assemble the pens, index cards, highlighters, post-it notes, and any other materials you may need so you won't be distracted by getting up to find things while you study.

If you're having a hard time retaining the information or organizing your notes, experiment with different methods. For example, try color-coding by subject with colored pens, highlighters, or post-it notes. If you learn better by hearing, try recording yourself reading your notes so you can listen while in the car, working out, or simply sitting at your desk. Ask a friend to quiz you from your flashcards, or try teaching someone the material to solidify it in your mind.

STEP 4: CREATE YOUR ENVIRONMENT

It's important to avoid distractions while you study. This includes both the obvious distractions like visitors and the subtle distractions like an uncomfortable chair (or a too-comfortable couch that makes you want to fall asleep). Set up the best study environment possible: good lighting and a comfortable work area. If background music helps you focus, you may want to turn it on, but otherwise keep the room quiet. If you are using a computer to take notes, be sure you don't have any other windows open, especially applications like social media, games, or anything else that could distract you. Silence your phone and turn off notifications. Be sure to keep water close by so you stay hydrated while you study (but avoid unhealthy drinks and snacks).

Also, take into account the best time of day to study. Are you freshest first thing in the morning? Try to set aside some time then to work through the material. Is your mind clearer in the afternoon or evening? Schedule your study session then. Another method is to study at the same time of day that you will take the test, so that your brain gets used to working on the material at that time and will be ready to focus at test time.

STEP 5: STUDY!

Once you have done all the study preparation, it's time to settle into the actual studying. Sit down, take a few moments to settle your mind so you can focus, and begin to follow your study plan. Don't give in to distractions or let yourself procrastinate. This is your time to prepare so you'll be ready to fearlessly approach the test. Make the most of the time and stay focused.

Of course, you don't want to burn out. If you study too long you may find that you're not retaining the information very well. Take regular study breaks. For example, taking five minutes out of every hour to walk briskly, breathing deeply and swinging your arms, can help your mind stay fresh.

As you get to the end of each chapter or section, it's a good idea to do a quick review. Remind yourself of what you learned and work on any difficult parts. When you feel that you've mastered the material, move on to the next part. At the end of your study session, briefly skim through your notes again.

But while review is helpful, cramming last minute is NOT. If at all possible, work ahead so that you won't need to fit all your study into the last day. Cramming overloads your brain with more information than it can process and retain, and your tired mind may struggle to recall even previously learned information when it is overwhelmed with last-minute study. Also, the urgent nature of cramming and the stress placed on your brain contribute to anxiety. You'll be more likely to go to the test feeling unprepared and having trouble thinking clearly.

So don't cram, and don't stay up late before the test, even just to review your notes at a leisurely pace. Your brain needs rest more than it needs to go over the information again. In fact, plan to finish your studies by noon or early afternoon the day before the test. Give your brain the rest of the day to relax or focus on other things, and get a good night's sleep. Then you will be fresh for the test and better able to recall what you've studied.

STEP 6: TAKE A PRACTICE TEST

Many courses offer sample tests, either online or in the study materials. This is an excellent resource to check whether you have mastered the material, as well as to prepare for the test format and environment.

Check the test format ahead of time: the number of questions, the type (multiple choice, free response, etc.), and the time limit. Then create a plan for working through them. For example, if you have 30 minutes to take a 60-question test, your limit is 30 seconds per question. Spend less time on the questions you know well so that you can take more time on the difficult ones.

If you have time to take several practice tests, take the first one open book, with no time limit. Work through the questions at your own pace and make sure you fully understand them. Gradually work up to taking a test under test conditions: sit at a desk with all study materials put away and set a timer. Pace yourself to make sure you finish the test with time to spare and go back to check your answers if you have time.

After each test, check your answers. On the questions you missed, be sure you understand why you missed them. Did you misread the question (tests can use tricky wording)? Did you forget the information? Or was it something you hadn't learned? Go back and study any shaky areas that the practice tests reveal.

Taking these tests not only helps with your grade, but also aids in combating test anxiety. If you're already used to the test conditions, you're less likely to worry about it, and working through tests until you're scoring well gives you a confidence boost. Go through the practice tests until you feel comfortable, and then you can go into the test knowing that you're ready for it.

Test Tips

On test day, you should be confident, knowing that you've prepared well and are ready to answer the questions. But aside from preparation, there are several test day strategies you can employ to maximize your performance.

First, as stated before, get a good night's sleep the night before the test (and for several nights before that, if possible). Go into the test with a fresh, alert mind rather than staying up late to study.

Try not to change too much about your normal routine on the day of the test. It's important to eat a nutritious breakfast, but if you normally don't eat breakfast at all, consider eating just a protein bar. If you're a coffee drinker, go ahead and have your normal coffee. Just make sure you time it so that the caffeine doesn't wear off right in the middle of your test. Avoid sugary beverages, and drink enough water to stay hydrated but not so much that you need a restroom break 10 minutes into the

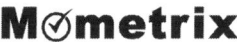

test. If your test isn't first thing in the morning, consider going for a walk or doing a light workout before the test to get your blood flowing.

Allow yourself enough time to get ready, and leave for the test with plenty of time to spare so you won't have the anxiety of scrambling to arrive in time. Another reason to be early is to select a good seat. It's helpful to sit away from doors and windows, which can be distracting. Find a good seat, get out your supplies, and settle your mind before the test begins.

When the test begins, start by going over the instructions carefully, even if you already know what to expect. Make sure you avoid any careless mistakes by following the directions.

Then begin working through the questions, pacing yourself as you've practiced. If you're not sure on an answer, don't spend too much time on it, and don't let it shake your confidence. Either skip it and come back later, or eliminate as many wrong answers as possible and guess among the remaining ones. Don't dwell on these questions as you continue—put them out of your mind and focus on what lies ahead.

Be sure to read all of the answer choices, even if you're sure the first one is the right answer. Sometimes you'll find a better one if you keep reading. But don't second-guess yourself if you do immediately know the answer. Your gut instinct is usually right. Don't let test anxiety rob you of the information you know.

If you have time at the end of the test (and if the test format allows), go back and review your answers. Be cautious about changing any, since your first instinct tends to be correct, but make sure you didn't misread any of the questions or accidentally mark the wrong answer choice. Look over any you skipped and make an educated guess.

At the end, leave the test feeling confident. You've done your best, so don't waste time worrying about your performance or wishing you could change anything. Instead, celebrate the successful completion of this test. And finally, use this test to learn how to deal with anxiety even better next time.

> **Review Video: Test Anxiety**
> Visit mometrix.com/academy and enter code: 100340

Important Qualification

Not all anxiety is created equal. If your test anxiety is causing major issues in your life beyond the classroom or testing center, or if you are experiencing troubling physical symptoms related to your anxiety, it may be a sign of a serious physiological or psychological condition. If this sounds like your situation, we strongly encourage you to seek professional help.

Online Resources

Due to our efforts to try to keep this book to a manageable length, we've created a link that will give you access to all of your online resources:

mometrix.com/resources719/cphq-27315

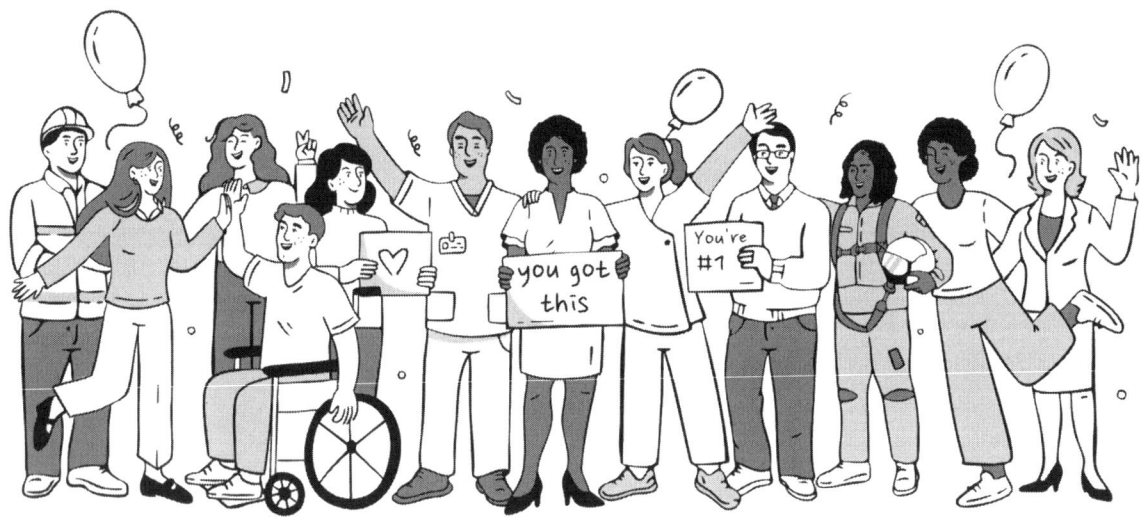